STUDY GUIDE

for the

Therapeutic Recreation Specialist Certification Examination

fourth edition

Norma J. Stumbo

Jean E. Folkerth

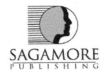

SAGAMORE
PUBLISHING

Publishers: Joseph J. Bannon and Peter L. Bannon
Director of Sales and Marketing: William A. Anderson
Director of Development and Production: Susan M. Davis
Technology Manager: Christopher Thompson
Production Coordinator: Amy S. Dagit

ISBN print edition: 978-1-57167- 716-7
ISBN ebook: 978-1-57167- 717-4
LCCN: 2012953041

Sagamore Publishing LLC
1807 N. Federal Dr.
Urbana, IL 61801
www.sagamorepub.com

CONTENTS

SECTION ONE

SECTION TWO

ABOUT THE AUTHORS

NORMA J. STUMBO received her B.S. and M.S. in Recreation and Park Administration/Therapeutic Recreation from the University of Missouri-Columbia and her Ph.D. in Leisure Studies/Therapeutic Recreation from the University of Illinois at Urbana-Champaign. She retired after serving as a professor and grant director at Illinois State University and the University of Illinois. Dr. Stumbo serves on the board of directors of the American Therapeutic Recreation Association (ATRA), serving as president-elect from 2012 to 2013, and president from 2013 to 2014. She also served on the board of directors of the National Council for Therapeutic Recreation Certification (NCTRC) from 1981 to 1989, serving as chair of the Test Management Committee from 1982 to 1989 and vice president from 1988 to 1989. She has authored over 160 publications, including *Facilitation of Therapeutic Recreation Services: An Evidence-Based and Best Practice Approach to Techniques and Processes*; *Therapeutic Recreation Program Design: Principles and Procedures*; *Client Assessment in Therapeutic Recreation Services*; *Client Outcomes in Therapeutic Recreation Services*; and *Professional Issues in Therapeutic Recreation Services: On Competence and Outcomes*, among others. She has conducted over 400 presentations at the local, state, national, and international levels, on a variety of topics, including client outcomes, evidence-based practice, entry-level knowledge, curriculum research, assessment, evaluation, and leisure education.

JEAN E. FOLKERTH received her B.S. in Camping and Outdoor Education/Therapeutic Recreation from Indiana University, her M.A. in Therapeutic Recreation from Michigan State University, and her Re.D. in Recreation Administration/Therapeutic Recreation from Indiana University. She retired from the University of Toledo after teaching over 27 years in higher education. Currently Dr. Folkerth works part time for the American Therapeutic Recreation Association as its academy coordinator and is responsible for ATRA's teleconference/webinar series and their newsletters. She continues to teach an occasional course and supervise interns for different universities. Dr. Folkerth served on the board of directors of the National Council for Therapeutic Recreation Certification from 1984 to 1989, serving as president from 1985 to 1987. She served on the board of directors of the National Therapeutic Recreation Society from 1979 to 1982 and was instrumental in the implementation of the State and Regional Advisory Council for NTRS. Dr. Folkerth has authored several publications and conducted over 100 presentations at state, regional, and national levels on topics including credentialing, professional preparation, and professional issues.

ACKNOWLEDGMENTS

Our many thanks to Dr. Nancy Navar, University of Wisconsin-LaCrosse in Wisconsin; Ray Archer, Stony Brook University Hospital in New York; Joseph Anderson, Grambling State University in Louisiana, and Renee Teshke from Grand Valley State University in Michigan for reviewing and providing extensive feedback on the practice test items.

We also owe thanks to the many individuals who used the previous editions and let us know what they thought about them. Their comments and questions have helped to improve the fourth edition. We hope the audience of the fourth edition feels equally free to share their advice about the *Study Guide*.

We would also like to acknowledge the assistance of Dr. Bob Riley, executive director of the National Council for Therapeutic Recreation Certification, who answered our lengthy list of questions about the exam and how it is administered.

We also appreciate the support of our friends, families, and partners.

The staff at Sagamore Publishing, once again, has been exceptional. We appreciate the support and enthusiasm of their efforts.

chapter 1

Introduction to the Study Guide

Welcome to the fourth edition of the *Study Guide for the Therapeutic Recreation Specialist Certification Examination*. We are excited to tell you that the fourth edition (2013) has changed significantly from previous editions in 2005, 1997, and 1990. This is largely due to two reasons: (a) the National Council for Therapeutic Recreation Certification (NCTRC) has recently updated the Job Analysis, which helps structure the content of the test, and (b) the computerized test has a newer format of a 90-item base test and 15-item testlets. Therefore, we have restructured the *Study Guide* to align more closely with the most recent NCTRC exam content and format.

As always, the absolute best information about the NCTRC exam comes directly from NCTRC. Candidates are encouraged to go directly to NCTRC for the most accurate, complete, and timely information. Candidates should not rely on other sources, such as word-of-mouth, colleagues, or unofficial websites or social media (such as Facebook) for correct information. Detailed information about the exam, such as when and where it is administered and sitting requirements in order to qualify for the exam, are available at:

National Council for Therapeutic Recreation Certification
7 Elmwood Drive
New City, NY 10956
Telephone: 845 639-1439
Fax: 845 639-1471
E-mail: nctrc@NCTRC.org
Website: www.NCTRC.org

Every test candidate is responsible for ensuring that he or she gets the best information available, directly from the National Office staff. Standards change periodically as do the test format and structure, so it is wise to check with the NCTRC staff to get the most accurate and timely information.

Purpose of the *Study Guide*

The purpose of this *Study Guide* is to assist candidates in preparing for the NCTRC national certification examination for Therapeutic Recreation Specialists. The *Study Guide*'s mission is twofold: (a) to provide information that helps candidates reduce test anxiety and maximize test performance and (b) to provide numerous sample questions, similar to those actually found on the exam, which will allow candidates to practice and self-assess their own readiness for the test.

We have tried to provide enough background information to give you some idea of what to expect when you take or "sit" for the exam. Every attempt has been made to make this *Study Guide* both usable and "user friendly." We hope you will find it both a valuable resource and a learning tool. This *Study Guide* is meant to be used in conjunction with, not as a replacement for, the *NCTRC Information for New Applicants,* one of the official documents found on the NCTRC website that provides very specific information about registering for and taking the national exam. In this *Study Guide* we do not address the sitting requirements or qualifications for taking the exam, as the candidate should go directly to NCTRC for that information. We do, however, cover the basics about the exam itself, and most importantly, provide over 700 items that are similar to the exam itself.

The *Study Guide* is divided into two basic sections. Section One of this *Study Guide* includes the following four chapters:

- Chapter One: Introduction to the Study Guide

- Chapter Two: Details about the NCTRC Exam

- Chapter Three: Strategies for Preparing and Taking the Test

- Chapter Four: Basic Information about the Test Content

Section Two of this *Study Guide* includes:

- Chapter Five:

  Warm-Up Items (160 items)

- Chapter Six:

  Practice Test 1 (90 items)

- Chapter Seven

  Practice Test 2 (90 items)

- Chapter Eight

  Practice Test 3 (90 items)

- Chapter Nine

  Practice Test 4 (90 items)

- Chapter Ten

  Practice Test 5 (90 items)

- Chapter Eleven

  Practice Test 6 (90 items)

A scoring sheet and a scoring key with the answers to each test are found at the end of each respective chapter.

How to Use the *Study Guide*

For many individuals, the thought of taking a certification examination can be unsettling. We often hear statements like, "I have never taken a comprehensive exam. There is so much information. How do I learn it all?" or "I've been out of school for ten years, how do I go about studying for the test?" Be assured that many of your colleagues across the nation have the same types of questions that you do. Hopefully, these kinds of questions and others will be answered by reading and completing this *Study Guide*.

We have tried to provide you with a condensed but complete set of materials. We trust that you will find the information and resources contained in the *Study Guide* helpful in getting ready for the national examination.

We advise that you read the first four chapters before going to the sample test questions. The beginning chapters in Section One provide important background information on the test and how to best prepare for it. Chapter Two covers basic information about the test such as number and distribution of items on the exam. This chapter contains the NCTRC Exam Content Outline, which forms the basis for the test. Chapter Three provides a variety of helpful hints in preparing for as well as taking the actual test. Chapter Four provides an extensive summary of the content presented on the exam, including useful references at the end of each section. Knowing this information can make the difference between passing or not passing the national examination.

The NCTRC Exam Content Outline, presented in both Chapters Two and Four, represents the result of several NCTRC committees working in conjunction with the Prometric testing company and lays the foundation for the examination. The Content Outline contains four areas that are represented on the test. **Study the Content Outline and accompanying information thoroughly.**

Before we go further, we want to clarify an important point. The format used for the items within this *Study Guide* is nearly identical to that used by NCTRC and Prometric to develop the national certification test. However, do not expect to see the same items on the actual NCTRC test. **The items in this Study Guide represent similar format and content as the NCTRC exam, but this does not mean they are the same items found on the test.** Keep in mind that these are practice items and that the authors of the *Study Guide* are not privy to the items on the exam.

In Section Two of the *Study Guide*, the sample test items are divided into seven chapters. Beyond the first chapter that contains 160 random practice items, each of the remaining chapters has a 90-item test that mirrors the base 90-item NCTRC examination. The 90 items are distributed across the Exam Content Outline in the same proportions as the official test. See Chapters Two and Four for more information on the Exam Content Outline.

If it has been a while since you have taken a multiple-choice test, take as many of these tests as you need to increase your comfort level. Familiarize yourself with the style of the items and get back into the feel of taking a test.

We suggest you sit and take each practice test in one sitting, to get the feel of how you will fare physically and mentally during the actual test. While we cannot copy the real testing environment, especially since the test is computerized, we want you to get a notion of how physical and mental fatigue may affect you. If this is significant, you may want to review the chapter on Strategies for Test Preparation.

A scoring sheet is provided at the end of each practice test chapter, as is a scoring key. The scoring keys should help you determine if you need more practice by taking additional tests. The scoring keys also provide more detailed diagnostic information about which parts of the Exam Content Outline you did well on, and which you did not. If there is one or more areas in which you did not do well, you may want to review the Exam Content Outline in Chapters Two and Four, especially the expanded content in Chapter 4 with references which may help your understanding of the material.

Again, we remind you that identical items will not be found on the actual NCTRC test. But if you find that you miss several items, say concerning documentation and goal writing, you will know this is an area on which you should concentrate your study efforts before you sit for the national exam.

Remember, the *Study Guide* is meant to be a framework to help you prepare for and to let you know what to expect on the test. You may use it as a diagnostic tool of sorts to learn the areas where you need more preparation.

chapter 2

Details about the NCTRC Exam

This chapter provides you with some details regarding the content and process of the NCTRC exam. Additional details are found in the *NCTRC Information for New Applicants* on the NCTRC website [www.nctrc.org].

During its last administration for which there is data (from October 2011 to May 2012), 1,528 individuals participated in the NCTRC program. The pass rate for these three administrations varied between 72 and 76%. Almost three-fourths of all individuals who sit for the exam, pass it on their first attempt. Approximately 3% of all individuals who recertify choose to take the exam as well, instead of pursuing the continuing education route (NCTRC, 2012).

Timing of the Exam

The NCTRC exam is administered by Prometric testing centers in the U.S., Canada, and Puerto Rico. The exam is offered three times per year, during a five-day period, in the months of January, May, and October. The candidate chooses the day of the week and time of day he or she takes the exam.

Variable Length Exam

The NCTRC exam is a variable length examination, meaning that there is a base test of 90 items, and depending on how you do, you may be given the option of taking additional items. You have up to 86 minutes to complete the 90-item base test.

At the end of the 90-item base test, you will receive a

a. passing score ending the exam,

b. failing score ending the exam, or

c. a score that falls in the range of neither failing nor passing.

If you received "c, a score that falls in the range of neither failing nor passing," you will move on to another section or "testlet."

Testlets are given one at a time, contain 15 items each, and are allowed 14 minutes each. At the end of *each* testlet you will once again receive a

a. passing score ending the exam,

b. failing score ending the exam, or

c. a score that falls in the range of neither passing nor failing.

You may be given from one to six testlets. Each testlet is proportional to the Exam Content Outline (see the section on Exam Content Outline later in this chapter).

Keep in mind that, like the base test, once you exit each testlet, you cannot go back. If you receive the base test and all six testlets of 15 items each, you will complete 180 test items and have a total of up to three hours of "seat time."

	# of Items	Minutes Allowed
Base Test	90	86
Testlet 1	15	14
Testlet 2	15	14
Testlet 3	15	14
Testlet 4	15	14
Testlet 5	15	14
Testlet 6	15	14
Total	180	170

Candidates need to think positively about the testlets if they become an option. Each testlet gives the test-taker a chance to prove what he or she knows. So instead of being dismayed by seeing a testlet start, the candidate should take a deep breath and see this as an opportunity to show what he or she knows.

Tutorial

Before starting the exam, candidates have the chance to take a brief, 10-minute tutorial to become more familiar with computerized testing. It is a nonscored tutorial that helps candidates become familiar with testing options, such as "Item Review," "Next," "Mark," and "Previous." If you have not ever nor recently taken a computerized test, it is a good idea to do this tutorial so your chances of making mistakes due to unfamiliarity with computerized testing are greatly lessened. You are given about 10 minutes to go through the tutorial. These 10 minutes are not subtracted from your time for your base test. Once you exit the tutorial, you cannot get back in it.

Special Arrangements

Test candidates with physical or cognitive disabilities who need reasonable accommodations during the exam need to contact NCTRC while they are being reviewed to sit for the exam to make special arrangements. These arrangements might include a reader, a marker/writer, a sign language interpreter, or extended time. Special accommodations cannot be made on-site without prior documentation and approval. All Prometric testing centers are required to comply with the Americans with Disabilities Act (ADA) regarding accessibility. Those individuals who have prior approval for testing accommodations need to call Prometric to schedule their test administration. The NCTRC office staff will help guide you through this process. Do make sure to give them adequate lead time so your needs can be accommodated.

About the Actual Test

While taking the test, you have the option of going back to previous items, and marking items without answering them so you can go back to them later. If you believe you might run short of time, it is a good idea to mark questions that you are unsure of, and answer those questions that you are most confident about. You can come back to the marked questions before you exit the exam, but do not forget to do so! Once you exit the exam, you cannot get back in.

There is no penalty for guessing at answers (like there is for other kinds of tests). Narrow down the options to those that are most likely to be right, and then choose which one you think is the best answer. If you are unsure, you can mark it and come back to the item later.

Exam Content Outline

The content of the exam is divided into four major areas:

(a) Foundational knowledge,

(b) Practice of therapeutic recreation,

(c) Organization of therapeutic recreation, and

(d) Advancement of the profession.

The 90-item base test (a combination of six 15-item testlets) as well as each additional 15-item testlet contains questions from these four areas in the same proportions. See the Table 1 for the number of items per testlet from each of the content areas.

Given the frequencies and percentages per testlet given in Table 1, the base 90-item test contains the distribution of questions found on Table 2.

Knowing the distribution of items across the four major exam content areas is important in that it can help focus your study. Candidates should concentrate on areas that (a) have the most items and (b) they are most unfamiliar with.

Table 3 provides an extended look at the Exam Content Outline. It provides more details about the content within each of the four major areas. You can compare the content of Table 3 with frequencies and percentages of test items under each heading on Table 1 to see how many items are in each area. For example, under the area of Foundational Knowledge, the sub-area of Background has one item per testlet or six items on the 90-item base test. On the base exam of 90 items, there will be six items from the Background area. Under the area of Foundational Knowledge, the sub-area of Diagnostic Groupings has 3 items per testlet or 18 items on the 90-item base test. On the base exam, there will be 18 items from the Diagnostic Groupings area. You can go through the Exam Content Outline and note how many items are within each of the headings. Use this information to concentrate your studies.

Table 1

NCTRC Exam Content and Item Percentages Per 15-Item Testlet (NCTRC, 2012)

Content Areas	Number of Test Items (Per Testlet)	Final Percentage
Foundational Knowledge	5	33.3%
A. Background	1	
B. Diagnostic Groupings	3	
C. Theories and Concepts	1	
Practice of TR/RT	7	46.7%
A. Strategies and Guidelines	1	
B. Assessment	2	
C. Documentation	2	
D. Implementation	2	
Organization of TR/RT	2	13.3%
A. TR Service Delivery	1	
B. Administrative Tasks	1	
Advancement of the Profession	1	16.7%
Total	**15**	**100.0%**

(The NCTRC® Certification Standards are the copyright property of, and used herein with permission from, the National Council for Therapeutic Recreation Certification®. All rights reserved 2012)

Table 2

Distribution of Items for the Base 90-Item NCTRC National Exam (NCTRC, 2012)

Content of Base Test	90 items
Foundational Knowledge	30
Practice of TR/RT	42
Organization of TR/RT	12
Advancement of Profession	6
Total =	**90 items**

(The NCTRC® Certification Standards are the copyright property of, and used herein with permission from, the National Council for Therapeutic Recreation Certification®. All rights reserved 2012)

Table 3

NCTRC Exam Content Outline (NCTRC, 2012)

I. Foundational Knowledge (30 items or 33.3% of the total test items)
  A. **Background (6 items)**
    1. Human growth and development throughout the lifespan
    2. Theories of human behavior and theories of behavior change
    3. Principles of behavioral change (e.g., self-efficacy theory, experiential learning model)
    4. Diversity factors (e.g., social, cultural, educational, language, spiritual, financial, age, attitude, geography)
    5. Concepts and models of health and human services (e.g., medical model, community model, education model, psychosocial rehabilitation model, health and wellness model, person-centered model, International Classification of Functioning {ICF})
    6. Principles of group interaction, leadership, and safety
  B. **Diagnostic Groupings (18 items)**
    1. Cognition and related impairments (e.g., dementia, traumatic brain injury, developmental/learning disabilities)
    2. Anatomy, physiology, and kinesiology and related impairments (e.g., impairments in musculoskeletal system, nervous system, circulatory system, respiratory system, endocrine system and metabolic disorders, infectious diseases)
    3. Senses and related impairments (e.g., vision, hearing)
    4. Psychology and related impairments (e.g., mental health, behavior, addictions)
  C. **Theories and Concepts (6 items)**
    1. Normalization, inclusion, and least restrictive environment
    2. Architectural barriers and accessibility
    3. Societal attitudes (e.g., stereotypes)
    4. Legislation (e.g., Americans with Disabilities Act, Older Americans Act)
    5. Relevant guidelines and standards (e.g. federal and state regulatory agencies)
    6. Theories of play, recreation, and leisure
    7. Social psychological aspects of play, recreation, and leisure
    8. Leisure throughout the lifespan
    9. Leisure lifestyle development

II. Practice of Therapeutic Recreation/Recreation Therapy (42 items or 46.7% of the total test items)
  A. **Strategies and Guidelines (6 items)**
    1. Concepts of TR/RT (e.g., holistic approach, recreative experience, special/adaptive recreation, inclusive recreation, using recreation as a treatment modality)
    2. Models of TR/RT service delivery (e.g., Leisure Ability Model, Health Protection/Health Promotion model, TR Service Delivery model)
    3. Practice settings (e.g., hospital, long-term care, community recreation, correctional facilities)
    4. Standards of practice for the TR/RT profession
    5. Code of ethics in the TR/RT field and accepted ethical practices with respect to culture, social, spiritual, and ethnic differences
  B. **Assessment (12 items)**
    1. Current TR/RT/leisure assessment instruments
    2. Other inventories and questionnaires (e.g., standardized ratings systems, developmental screening tests, MDS, GIM, GAF)
    3. Other sources of assessment data (e.g., records or charts, staff, support system)
    4. Criteria for selection and/or development of assessment (e.g., purpose, reliability, validity, practicality, availability)
    5. Implementation of assessment
    6. Behavioral observations related to assessment
    7. Interview techniques for assessment

8. Functional skills testing for assessment
9. Sensory assessment (e.g., vision, hearing, tactile)
10. Cognitive assessment (e.g., memory, problem solving, attention span, orientation, safety awareness)
11. Social assessment (e.g., communication/interactive skills, relationships)
12. Physical assessment (e.g., fitness, motor skills function)
13. Affective assessment (e.g., attitude toward self, expression)
14. Leisure assessment (e.g., barriers, interests, values, patterns/skills, knowledge)

D. Documentation (12 items)
1. Impact of impairment and/or treatment on the person served (e.g., side effects of medications, medical precautions)
2. Interpretation of assessment and record of person served
3. Documentation of assessment, progress/functional status, discharge/transition plan of person served (e.g., SOAP, FIM)
4. Methods of writing measurable goals and behavioral objectives

E. Implementation (12 items)
1. Nature and diversity of recreation and leisure activities
2. Selection of programs, activities, and interventions to achieve the assessed needs of the person served
3. Purpose and techniques of activity/task analysis
4. Activity modifications (e.g., assistive techniques, technology and adaptive devices, rule changes)
5. Modalities and/or interventions (e.g., therapeutic recreation/recreation therapy activities, leisure skill development, assertiveness training, stress management, social skills, community reintegration)
6. Facilitation techniques and/or approaches (e.g., behavior management, counseling skills)
7. Leisure education/counseling

III. Organization of Therapeutic Recreation/Recreation Therapy Service (12 items or 13.3% of the total test items)

A. TR Service Design (6 items)
1. Program design relative to population served
2. Type of service delivery systems (e.g., health, leisure services, education and human services)
3. Role and function of other health and human service professions and of interdisciplinary approaches
4. Documentation procedures for program accountability, and payment for services
5. Methods for interpretation of progress notes, observations, and assessment results of the person being served

B. Administrative Tasks (6 items)
1. Evaluating agency or TR/RT service program
2. Quality improvement guidelines and techniques (e.g., utilization review, risk management, peer review, outcome monitoring)
3. Components of agency or TR/RT service plan of operation
4. Personnel, intern, and volunteer supervision and management
5. Payment system (e.g., managed care, PPO, private contract, Medicare, Medicaid, DRG)
6. Facility and equipment management
7. Budgeting and fiscal responsibility

IV. Advancement of the Profession (6 items or 6.7% of the total test items)
1. Historical development of TR/RT
2. Accreditation standards and regulations (e.g., JCAHO, CARF, CMS)
3. Professionalism (professional behavior and professional development)
4. Requirements for TR/RT credentialing (e.g., certification, recertification, licensure)
5. Advocacy for persons served
6. Legislation and regulations pertaining to TR/RT
7. Professional standards and ethical guidelines pertaining to the TR/RT profession
8. Public relations, promotion, and marketing of the TR/RT profession
9. Methods, resources, and references for maintaining and upgrading professional competencies
10. Professional associations and organizations

11. Partnerships between higher education and direct service providers to provide internships and to produce, understand, and interpret research for advancement of the TR/RT profession
12. Value of continuing education and in-service training for the advancement of the TR/RT profession

(The NCTRC® Certification Standards are the copyright property of, and used herein with permission from, the National Council for Therapeutic Recreation Certification®. All rights reserved 2012)

Test Scoring

The exam is based on a cut score, the dividing line between those who pass the test or do not pass the test. You will not receive a score (say, 70% or a "C"). You will receive an unofficial notification of whether or not you passed the exam, on the computer screen immediately at the end of your session. Official notification will be sent by Prometric within a couple of weeks, after the end of the testing week in which you took your exam.

If you pass, the notification will indicate that. If you do not pass, you will receive a 'scaled score' between 20 and 54. In addition, you will be given feedback, based on each of the four areas of the Exam Content Outline. For each of the four areas, you will receive a 1, indicat-ing that your score in that area was below the minimum competency expected, or a 2, indicating your score was at or above the minimal acceptable level for that area. This feedback is provided so you may focus your study and efforts for the next time you take the exam. If you do not pass, you may register for the next available test.

All NCTRC tests are comprised of a 90-item base and possible 15-item testlets. Should you need to take the exam more than once, you will be re-tested on all material covered in the Exam Content Outline, regardless of how you did on prior tests. If you take the exam subsequent times, you need to prepare for the entire scope of content, focusing specifically on the areas that you did not do well during prior tests.

chapter 3

Strategies for Preparing for and Taking the Test

This chapter of the *Study Guide* is divided into two major sections: preparing for the test and taking the test. Each section contains helpful hints to assist you while you are studying and sitting for the exam. The exam consists entirely of four-answer-option, multiple-choice questions, and these strategies are based on that fact.

Overall, one major way to improve your test score is to become as familiar as possible with the test content. Read the Exam Content Outline (see Table 3 in Chapter Two and Table 1 in Chapter 4) thoroughly. Use the sample items found in the practice tests to practice and self-diagnose your weaker areas.

The second major way to improve your test score is to improve your test taking skills. That is, becoming more "test wise." Often, a person's score may be reduced simply because he or she makes errors in recording answers, eliminating wrong answer options, and leaving questions blank. While the other sections of this Study Guide attempt to help you become familiar with the test content, this section deals exclusively with reviewing test-taking strategies, helping you become more "test wise."

The hint you might find most helpful in this process is to relax and enjoy it as much as possible. If nothing else, you will exit the testing center knowing just a bit more about the profession than when you entered, and that benefits everyone.

Preparing for the Test

1. **Start early.** If possible, give yourself at least one to two months to study before taking the exam. This time can be used for reviewing the job analysis and content outline information, looking up new or un-

familiar information, ordering necessary materials, and reviewing your notes.

2. Review *Part I: Information for New Applicants*, **available on the NCTRC website [www.nctrc.org.].** This document has all the current information about the exam, including the sitting requirements, etc. Become as familiar as possible with this document so you understand clearly what the test contains and how it is administered.

3. **Review the knowledge areas within the Content Outline and complete the sample test questions.** If you have concerns about your comprehension in any area, review thoroughly the overview of the exam content provided in Chapter Four. Use the reference list at the end of each section to identify which resources you have and which you may need to obtain. Notice which references are used repeatedly and look at those first.

4. **Do not assume that you know everything about the knowledge areas that is necessary, based on your performance on these sample questions.** We have provided the questions for your practice, but they are not exhaustive or definitive of the material covered on the exam. It is quite likely that you will encounter a question or two on the exam that cover content that is unfamiliar to you, such as s specific practice setting or diagnostic information or regulatory standards. Knowing that you are likely to encounter such items will help you deal with them when the time comes.

4. **Determine how you study best.** Some individuals seem to learn better when they hear the information, while others need to see written materials, and still others prefer to discuss material with colleagues. A combination of these alternatives often can produce the most effective study patterns. We suggest you review the material individually, and then use groups of colleagues for discussion and brainstorming of material.

5. **Create your own review materials.** This might be in the form of an outline, note cards, flash cards, etc. As you make your own learning materials, you will find that this helps you learn the material more deeply. For example, you might copy the Exam Content Outline on sheets of paper, then search for information, and jot it down under each area. Or prepare a note card or two for each knowledge area, and then under each heading list relevant information as thoughtfully and concisely as possible. It also may help you to keep track of reference materials on the outline or note cards so if questions arise later, you will be able to track down the information more quickly.

6. **Concentrate your study efforts by prioritizing what you need to study.** If you have not opened a textbook or journal for some time, this is not the time to try to catch up and read all the available material. Concentrate on a few well-chosen references from the reference list. Note there are some references that are used repeatedly throughout Chapter Four. Also concentrate on the knowledge areas that have been listed as most important to practice, according to the Exam Content Outline (Table 3 in Chapter Two and Table 1 in Chapter 4).

   These content areas are the focal point for the exam content and should provide direction for your study sessions. Remember to look at the percentages of weight for each area, to know how many questions will be asked per area.

7. **Network, network, network!** Do not hesitate to call on colleagues. Use them both as content experts and as study partners to discuss the content covered by the test. This will be helpful to all parties. Perhaps your study group might contain colleagues who work with a variety of populations in various settings. You might find it helpful to compare the practice of therapeutic recreation in diverse settings applied to different populations. Do remember to look for similarities rather than differences in practice. The job analysis revealed that there was overwhelming consensus on the sub-categories of the knowledge areas so material applicable across settings will

be most useful to review. Your group may also find it helpful to create your own sample test items and review them as a group.

8. **Use whatever test anxiety you may have positively instead of negatively.** Use this energy to make the test a positive, rather than negative, experience. Think of the benefits of updating and reviewing your knowledge and focus on the larger picture of competent practice. Always ask yourself, "How does this information apply to practice? How can I use this information to benefit my clients? How can I use this information in the future?" The more you can concentrate your efforts in creating a positive mental state, instead of a negative one, the better off you will be.

9. **Approach the test cognitively rather than emotionally.** The more you know about the content and percentages, as well as how the test is administered, the more you can approach the test cognitively rather than emotionally. Take time to read *Part I: Information for New Applicants* [www.NCTRC.org] as well as the entirety of this *Study Guide* so that you will know what to expect and not be taken off guard.

9. **If you have a physical or cognitive disability that requires accommodation, contact the NCTRC office prior to signing up for the test.** Prometric testing centers are required to meet local and federal guidelines for accessibility, but typical accommodations might include a reader, a separate room, extended examination time, etc., based on a documented disability. Contact the NCTRC office for complete details on asking for reasonable accommodations for a documented disability.

10. **Eat sensibly and get plenty of rest the night before the test to make sure you are at your physical best.** Make sure you get a good night's sleep ahead of the test. Also be sure to eat a sensible meal or snack before entering the testing center, as the test may take you anywhere from 30 minutes to three hours of "seat" time in addition to the time it takes to get processed at the center. Dress comfortably, perhaps in layers, so that you can adjust to the temperature of the room if you need to.

11. **Your absolute best strategy is to be as prepared as possible for the test.** We recommend three preparation materials: (a) NCTRC offers a 15-item practice test for free on their website; (b) NCTRC offers a 60-item practice test for a fee ($24.95); and (c) this *Study Guide*.

12. **This *Study Guide* is only a start; your thorough preparation is up to you.** You know best how much and what kinds of studying are most beneficial to you. It is probably better to be a bit overprepared than underprepared. Study well in advance, feel confident with your level of knowledge, and then relax.

Taking the Test

1. **Arrive at your test site at least 30 minutes early and do not forget to allow time for parking or finding the building/room.** Do not bring friends or relatives with you as they will not be allowed to sit in the waiting room while you are taking the exam.

2. **When you arrive at the testing site the following activities will occur:**
   a. You will be asked to present your ATT (the clearance form that you receive in the mail from Prometric) and photo-bearing identification that also has your signature (Check NCTRC's information for acceptable forms of ID).
   b. You will be asked to sign in at the center and that signature will be compared to the presented identification.
   c. Any and all belongings will be held in a secure locker prior to entering the testing area. Do not bring any drinks, food, paper, notebooks, backpacks, laptops, cell phones, etc. with you. You will not be allowed to bring any items into the testing room other than your identification.

3. **You will then be escorted to a computer terminal.** The test administrator will give you a packet of scratch paper that you may use as needed. It must be given to the test administrator when you leave.

4. **A brief online tutorial to guide you on how to use the computer for the exam will be provided.** The tutorial will familiarize you with selecting answers, using the testing features, using the mouse, and the overall operation of the keyboard. The tutorial is a "one-time deal." Make sure you understand how to mark the answers and operate the system because once you exit the tutorial, you may not return to it.

5. **Read each test question carefully.** For each question, study the statement of the question (or item stem). Before you look at the four multiple-choice options, try to answer the question in your own words. Then look at the choices very carefully, not trying to find out what is right about them, but studying them to find what is wrong. Eliminate all choices that are obviously wrong or implausible, and there should always be one choice that is either ob-viously correct or that is the least wrong. Do make sure you read through all the answer options; do not select the first one that sounds appropriate. For example, even if option A sounds correct, be sure to read through options B, C, and D. Choose the best possible answer for that question. All items have four answer options (A, B, C, D).

There will be no trick questions on the test, so try not to "read too much" into a question. For example, if a question concerns individuals with dementia, do not "add" other content to the question than what is there; don't add conditions or characteristics that are not part of the question. Prometric and NCTRC have stated each question as concisely as possible and give you all the information you need to select the best answer.

6. **Bypass those questions that you are unsure of, marking them as a reminder to review them later.** You are able to move back and forth within the base test, but the base test may not be reentered once it has been exited. Do not go back and reconsider marked answers, trying to second guess your first-choice answers. Most likely you were right the first time and will be changing a correct answer.

Do know that you may be unfamiliar with some of the content or items found on the test. Of course you don't want this to happen too frequently, but if you know ahead of time that you are likely to come across an item or two that you do not know, it will help you to answer the item the best you can and then move on.

7. **Eliminate as many answer options as possible.** As you read through each item and the four answer options, try to eliminate as many of the answers that you know are wrong. For example, after reading an item stem and all four responses, you know that option D is clearly wrong. Eliminating that answer option increases your chances of answering correctly, from 25% (evenly distributed through all four answer options) to 33% (evenly distributed through three answer options). If you can eliminate one more answer option, with two remaining, that brings you to a 50% chance of being correct!

8. **Pace yourself.** The base test consists of 90 questions for which you have 86 minutes. This is plenty of time to easily complete the test. For best results, pace yourself by periodically checking your progress. Set a pace that will allow you to make any necessary adjustments to unanswered questions. Work as quickly as you can without being careless.

9. **Be sure to record an answer for each question, even the ones you are not completely confident of.** Make informed guesses rather than leaving items unanswered. Eliminate as many alternatives as possible on multiple-choice items before guessing. There will be no penalty for guessing.

10. **Throughout the test, remind yourself to combat any emotional responses with self-statements, such as: "Just relax; I am in control; concentrate on doing well on this exam."** Sometimes we are our own worst critic, and in a testing situation this self-criticism may have a more negative than positive effect.

11. **Do your best but don't stress!** If you have studied well and prepared ahead of time, you should be able to relax the day of the exam. Take a deep breath and do the best you can.

References

Anatasi, A. (1954). *Psychological testing.* New York: MacMillan.

Bergmen, J. (1981). *Understanding educational measurement and evaluation.* Boston, MA: Houghton Mifflin.

Drummond, R. J. (1988). *Appraisal procedures for counselors and helping professionals.* Columbus, OH: Merrill.

Kaplan, R. M., & Saccuzzo, D. P. (1982). *Psychological testing: Principles, applications and issues.* Monterey, CA: Brooks Cole.

National Council for Therapeutic Recreation Certification. (2012). *Part I: Information for New Applicants.* Available at: www.nctrc.org

chapter 4

Basic Information on the Test Content Outline

The purpose of this chapter is to provide more detailed information about the content that will be on the national certification test. This section will act as a guide through the four different NCTRC Knowledge Areas. Its intent is to clarify concepts and to provide resources that may help you study more effectively and be better prepared for the national exam. If at the end of each section you feel you need more information, there is a list of resources that can be used to review a specific concept more thoroughly.

Introduction

The original NCTRC job analysis project results in 1989-1990 presented information about nine major job responsibilities and eight major knowledge areas. The last job analysis caused some major shifting and re-categorizing but content essentially remained the same. The knowledge areas were reduced to four. The primary changes occurred in the number of items on the test and the percentage weights of each topic. There was minimal change in the overall content, although some shifting and updating of areas occurred.

The job analysis essentially is the blueprint for the development of the national exam. That is, the test was developed based on this content outline. Table 1 presents the prevalence of test items on each of the four areas of the 90-item test.

Table 1

Distribution of Items for the Base NCTRC National Exam (NCTRC, 2012)

Content of Base Test	90 items
Foundational Knowledge	30
Practice of TR/RT	42
Organization of TR/RT	12
Advancement of Profession	6
Total =	**90 items**

Table 2 presents the NCTRC Exam Content Outline that is used as a guide for the remainder of this chapter. It also establishes a basis for reviewing the material covered within each category as well as providing general references for concepts and material. At the end of this chapter is a recommended reference list with ISBN numbers included, so materials can be ordered directly from the publisher if they cannot be located at your local or university library or bookstore. This reference list contains books that were used most frequently in this chapter.

Table 2

NCTRC Exam Content Outline (NCTRC, 2012)

I. Foundational Knowledge (30 items or 33.3% of the total test items)

A. Background (6 items)
1. Human growth and development throughout the lifespan
2. Theories of human behavior and theories of behavior change
3. Principles of behavioral change (e.g., self-efficacy theory, experiential learning model)
4. Diversity factors (e.g., social, cultural, educational, language, spiritual, financial, age, attitude, geography)
5. Concepts and models of health and human services (e.g., medical model, community model, education model, psychosocial rehabilitation model, health and wellness model, person-centered model, International Classification of Functioning {ICF})
6. Principles of group interaction, leadership, and safety

B. Diagnostic Groupings (18 items)
1. Cognition and related impairments (e.g., dementia, traumatic brain injury, developmental/learning disabilities)
2. Anatomy, physiology, and kinesiology and related impairments (e.g., impairments in musculoskeletal system, nervous system, circulatory system, respiratory system, endocrine system and metabolic disorders, infectious diseases)
3. Senses and related impairments (e.g., vision, hearing)
4. Psychology and related impairments (e.g., mental health, behavior, addictions)

C. Theories and Concepts (6 items)
1. Normalization, inclusion, and least restrictive environment
2. Architectural barriers and accessibility
3. Societal attitudes (e.g., stereotypes)
4. Legislation (e.g., Americans with Disabilities Act, Older Americans Act)
5. Relevant guidelines and standards (e.g. federal and state regulatory agencies)
6. Theories of play, recreation, and leisure
7. Social psychological aspects of play, recreation, and leisure
8. Leisure throughout the lifespan
9. Leisure lifestyle development

II. Practice of Therapeutic Recreation/Recreation Therapy (42 items or 46.7% of the total test items)

A. Strategies and Guidelines (6 items)
1. Concepts of TR/RT (e.g., holistic approach, recreative experience, special/adaptive recreation, inclusive recreation, using recreation as a treatment modality)
2. Models of TR/RT service delivery (e.g., Leisure Ability Model, Health Protection/Health Promotion model, TR Service Delivery model)
3. Practice settings (e.g., hospital, long-term care, community recreation, correctional facilities)
4. Standards of practice for the TR/RT profession
5. Code of ethics in the TR/RT field and accepted ethical practices with respect to culture, social, spiritual, and ethnic differences

B. Assessment (12 items)
1. Current TR/RT/leisure assessment instruments
2. Other inventories and questionnaires (e.g., standardized ratings systems, developmental screening tests, MDS, GIM, GAF)
3. Other sources of assessment data (e.g., records or charts, staff, support system)
4. Criteria for selection and/or development of assessment (e.g., purpose, reliability, validity, practicality, availability)
5. Implementation of assessment
6. Behavioral observations related to assessment
7. Interview techniques for assessment

8. Functional skills testing for assessment
9. Sensory assessment (e.g., vision, hearing, tactile)
10. Cognitive assessment (e.g., memory, problem solving, attention span, orientation, safety awareness)
11. Social assessment (e.g., communication/interactive skills, relationships)
12. Physical assessment (e.g., fitness, motor skills function)
13. Affective assessment (e.g., attitude toward self, expression)
14. Leisure assessment (e.g., barriers, interests, values, patterns/skills, knowledge)

D. Documentation (12 items)
1. Impact of impairment and/or treatment on the person served (e.g., side effects of medications, medical precautions)
2. Interpretation of assessment and record of person served
3. Documentation of assessment, progress/functional status, discharge/transition plan of person served (e.g., SOAP, FIM)
4. Methods of writing measurable goals and behavioral objectives

E. Implementation (12 items)
1. Nature and diversity of recreation and leisure activities
2. Selection of programs, activities, and interventions to achieve the assessed needs of the person served
3. Purpose and techniques of activity/task analysis
4. Activity modifications (e.g., assistive techniques, technology and adaptive devices, rule changes)
5. Modalities and/or interventions (e.g., therapeutic recreation/recreation therapy activities, leisure skill development, assertiveness training, stress management, social skills, community reintegration)
6. Facilitation techniques and/or approaches (e.g., behavior management, counseling skills)
7. Leisure education/counseling

III. Organization of Therapeutic Recreation/Recreation Therapy Service (12 items or 13.3% of the total test items)

A. TR Service Design (6 items)
1. Program design relative to population served
2. Type of service delivery systems (e.g., health, leisure services, education and human services)
3. Role and function of other health and human service professions and of interdisciplinary approaches
4. Documentation procedures for program accountability, and payment for services
5. Methods for interpretation of progress notes, observations, and assessment results of the person being served

B. Administrative Tasks (6 items)
1. Evaluating agency or TR/RT service program
2. Quality improvement guidelines and techniques (e.g., utilization review, risk management, peer review, outcome monitoring)
3. Components of agency or TR/RT service plan of operation
4. Personnel, intern, and volunteer supervision and management
5. Payment system (e.g., managed care, PPO, private contract, Medicare, Medicaid, DRG)
6. Facility and equipment management
7. Budgeting and fiscal responsibility

IV. Advancement of the Profession (6 items or 6.7% of the total test items)
1. Historical development of TR/RT
2. Accreditation standards and regulations (e.g., JCAHO, CARF, CMS)
3. Professionalism (professional behavior and professional development)
4. Requirements for TR/RT credentialing (e.g., certification, recertification, licensure)
5. Advocacy for persons served
6. Legislation and regulations pertaining to TR/RT
7. Professional standards and ethical guidelines pertaining to the TR/RT profession
8. Public relations, promotion, and marketing of the TR/RT profession
9. Methods, resources, and references for maintaining and upgrading professional competencies
10. Professional associations and organizations

11. Partnerships between higher education and direct service providers to provide internships and to produce, understand, and interpret research for advancement of the TR/RT profession

12. Value of continuing education and in-service training for the advancement of the TR/RT profession

I. Foundational Knowledge
(30 items or 33.3% of the total test items)

This knowledge area is to ensure that the entry-level professional has an understanding of the background, diagnostic groups, and theoretical and conceptual basis of information that pertains directly to therapeutic recreation. Most of the information for this section will come from support courses and recreation courses.

A. Background
1. Human Growth and Development

Understanding *human growth and development* is an important aspect of therapeutic recreation. Having a general understanding of a person's general growth and development (cognitive, physical, emotional, and social) helps to establish realistic expectations of clients and to provide appropriate interventions and treatment plans. The following material is very generic and does not try to cover all the changes that occur during a life stage.

Early childhood consists of those ages between birth and around six. During this time a child should be developing fundamental motor skills and social skills; a child's body is changing rapidly, and most children are very interested in finding out what exactly their limits are cognitively, physically, socially, and emotionally. Communication skills are also developing. Play is very important for children of these ages, for it is through play that many of their skills are developed and enhanced.

Children are those between the ages of six and 12. During this time the child's social world expands; he or she begins to be involved in organized sports, games, and extracurricular activities such as dance classes and music lessons. Children are still very involved in play, and their hand/eye coordination is improving. As the child grows older, friends become more significant than family and being like everyone else becomes very important.

Adolescence is the next stage and covers the ages between 13 and 21, approximately. This is the time when peer groups (peer pressure) become more important than family, and an individual struggles to become more independent from the family. The body begins to reach maturation and the interest in intimate relationships increases. Sexuality becomes intense with hormones influencing behavior. Organized sports, music, and the "mall" may become very important. Individuals are usually beginning to define themselves in their own right (e.g., as athletes or perhaps scholars). Peer groups continue to be important, but by the end of older adolescence, family is regaining its importance.

Individuals in the early adulthood stages (ages 21-30) usually establish their independence by completing their education and seeking their own occupation. During this time, they may begin to have more serious intimate relationships in order to establish families of their own. Their bodies have reached maturation, and the interest may be on more challenging leisure activities such as rock climbing or other activities that allow for the growth of relationships, such as movies and dinners. This is also the time when a person may develop an interest in more life-long leisure pursuits, such as golf, tennis, or running.

The years between 30 and 45 are known as middle adulthood. A person's family and career take priority. During this period many adults find themselves actively involved in their children's leisure pursuits. They attend sporting activities, concerts, plays, etc., and volunteer as coaches and leaders for various youth organizations. Their activities may be very family oriented, such as game nights, family vacations, etc. Occasionally, the person is involved in individual pursuits such as golf or running.

Older adulthood occurs approximately between the ages of 45 and 60. For most people there is a slowing down, and as the metabolism begins to change, there is a weight gain. Physical abilities also change with reductions in strength and flexibility. Cognitively, however, skills, and abilities remain strong. This is the life stage where people may experience midlife crises and depression. Children have moved out and the parents of people in this life stage are becoming dependent. It can be a very stressful time in life, yet it can also be very freeing when parents are still healthy and their own children are having children and advancing in their own careers.

Senior adulthood is the stage between 60 and 75. Most people have great amounts of free time and are retired. Although many individuals are beginning to experience health problems, most individuals are healthy, vigorous, and have the freedom to travel and participate in activities of their choosing.

The "old-old" stage occurs from age 75 to death. For some people, physical deterioration is rapid, and for others it is cognitive deterioration that seems to occur rapidly. The vast majority of people in this age group will experience health problems and need assistance. Their world may become smaller due to the death of friends and the need to live in a facility that can provide the assistance they need. Although many people will be limited in their abilities, there are others who will continue to be active (Edginton, Jordan, De-Graf, & Edginton, 2002; Feil, 1993; Godbey, 2003; Jordan, 2001; Russell, 2001).

2. Theories of Human Behavior and Theories of Behavior Change

It is assumed that entry-level professionals will understand *theories of human behavior and theories of behavior change.*

At this time, the largest population served by therapeutic recreation specialists is in behavioral health. There are four major theories of helping that apply to behavioral health that may be the underlying philosophy of an agency. The four theories are psychoanalytic, behavioristic, growth or positive psychology and cognitive-behavioral.

Psychoanalytic therapy was developed by Sigmund Freud and is based on the influence of instincts on thought and behavior. Freud believes that "there exists within each person a basic tendency to allow the maximum gratification of the primitive instincts, while giving minimum attention to the demands of society" (Austin, 2009, p. 11). Freud proposed a balance model identifying three divisions of personality: id, ego, and superego. Freud focused a lot of attention on the sexual instinct and proposed five psychosexual stages: oral, anal, phallic, latency, and genital. Freud also formulated defense mechanisms used by the ego: denial, repression, displacement, projection, sublimation, rationalization, and intellectualization. According to Austin (2009), "Recreational therapists must recognize that unconscious motivational factors may affect behavior, the use of defense mechanisms in protecting against threats to self-concept, and the effects the developmental years have on adult behavior" (p. 20).

Behavioristic theory is often referred to as behavior modification. Several well-known psychologists have developed theories and principles associated with behavior therapy. Pavlov's classical condition involves the principle of association and Thorndike's instrumental conditioning involves the principle of reinforcement. Essentially behaviorists believe that behavior is learned, so abnormal behavior has been learned, thus it can be changed (Austin, 2009).

Humanistic behavior sees people as "being self-aware, capable of accepting or rejecting environmental influences and generally in conscious control of their own destiny" (Austin, 2009, p. 31). Carl Rogers developed person-centered therapy. He stated that the therapist must demonstrate an unconditional positive regard for the client; that techniques are secondary to how the therapist treats the client. Many of the beliefs of Rogers are taught in therapeutic recreation courses to develop open communication with clients. Also included in this category is reality therapy and gestalt therapy.

Probably the most widely accepted method of behavioral change is the cognitive behavioral change process. It is based on the premise that "a person's thoughts or cognitions, dictate how he or she reacts emotionally and behaviorally to any particular situation" (Long, 2011, p. 289) There are essentially three components to this principle. The first component is "antecedents" which are the thoughts, perceptions, or beliefs that a person has about a topic or experience. The second component is "action" which is the actual behavior of the patient or client. The last component is "consequences," which refers to the actual response to the action. This response can reinforce the original thoughts, beliefs, or perceptions. The client will have specific beliefs or thoughts, and perceptions (antecedents) about something and behave in a way that displays those antecedents. The therapeutic recreation specialist will use a structured therapeutic recreation intervention that will have an impact on the outcome thus influencing the consequences (Austin, 2009; Dattilo & Murphy, 1987; Long, 2011; Shank & Coyle, 2002).

3. Principles of Behavioral Change

Principles of behavioral change also include self-efficacy, the attribution model, and the concept of learned helplessness. The entry-level professional needs to understand not only the concepts, but also how clients/patients might display these behaviors. When a person displays self-efficacy, essentially he or she is demonstrating the expectations of his or her ability to cope with his or her problems. A person must be confident of his or her abilities and not give up when the results of his or her actions are not immediate. If a person has recently become a paraplegic and is able to begin thinking of changes in his or her leisure activities (i.e., the adaptations necessary, trying them out, and not giving up when the results are not perfect), the person is beginning to cope and probably has good self-efficacy.

The attribution model deals with a person's explanation of the cause of events that occurred in that person's life. A person may explain the event due to internal or external attributes. For example, a client might believe that he was fired due to the "boss's dislike of him," which is an "external attribute," rather than his not completing tasks on time, which would be an "internal attribute." Understanding what attributes the client assigns to events will help the therapist work with the client. Helping the client to understand his role in an event is very important for the client's growth.

Learned helplessness is another theory of behavior change that the entry-level professional needs to understand. According to Mannell and Kleiber (1997), learned helplessness is "the phenomenon in which experience with uncontrollable events creates passive behavior toward subsequent threats to well-being" (p. 134). For example, when a client experiences consistent failure in physical activities as a child, she may refuse to try new physical activities as an adult because of that early failure, or she may try them but put little effort in achieving success because of her belief that she will not succeed.

The Transtheoretical Model "examines an individual's motivation and readiness to modify a particular behavior" (Stumbo & Pegg, 2011, p. 126). It suggests there are five major steps to change: pre-contemplation, contemplation, decision, action, and maintenance. The Theory of Reasoned Action/ Planned Behavior, one of the most recognized theories, looks at a person's attitudes toward a behavior, his or her perceptions of norms and beliefs about how easy or difficult it will be to change. Looking at various models and understanding them will help the entry level therapist especially in dealing with persons in healthcare (Austin, 2009; Iso-Ahola, 1980; Mannell & Kleiber, 1997; Shank & Coyle, 2002; Stumbo & Pegg, 2011).

4. Diversity Factors

In many ways the United States is becoming a more diverse nation. With this *diversity*, we recognize that many cultures and socioeconomic groups make up our country. As a result there are "pockets" of cultural differences in relation to beliefs about recreation, leisure, and disability. It is important that the entry-level therapist understands and respects those differences. Thus, along with understanding the impact of various life stages, it is important to have an understanding of the impact of diversity because it can increase the benefits of the treatment process. There are five primary dimensions of diversity that generate the strongest emotional response: race and ethnicity, gender, physical impairments and qualities, sexual orientation, and age. Secondary characteristics impact judgments about people as further interaction takes place. These include: economic status, religion, military experience, education, geographic location, marital status, parental status, and type of job (Getz, 2002).

5. Models of Health Care and Human Services

Knowing the *models of health care and human services* is another competency found under the topic of Background. As an entry-level professional, you need to have an understanding of the medical model, since many hospitals utilize this model. Also the psychosocial rehabilitation model is used in many healthcare facilities. Health and wellness have grown and become a function of many healthcare facilities. Thus, you need to have a basic understanding of these models. The person-centered model seems to be the model that is used by therapeutic recreation personnel in all areas of service. The most recently added model is the International Classification of Functioning, Disability and Health (ICF). The ICF was established by the World Health Organization (WHO) in an effort to "describe holistic health and to make possible a worldwide system of standardized communication and collaboration in health care. ...The ICF is an interactive model that illustrates the relationship between the concepts of a person's health condition, body structures and body functions activities and participation, and environmental and personal factors" (Howard, Dieser, Yang, Pegg & Lammel, 2008, p. 232-233). The ICF is very compatible with therapeutic recreation due to its focus on body function, activities and participation (Carter & van Andel, 2011; Howard et al., 2008; Porter & Burlingame, 2006).

6. Principles of Group Interaction and Leadership

The last competency in this knowledge area is *principles of group interaction and leadership*. Being able to lead group intervention sessions is very important in the field of therapeutic recreation. Because many of our activities take place within groups, the entry-level therapist needs to have an understanding of groups. According to Shank and Coyle (2002), "...groups provide opportunities for interactions among clients, and recreation therapists use these interactions to facilitate therapeutic outcomes" (p. 211). Thus having an understanding of group structure, principles, and leadership is important. There are important structural elements in a group: size, format (closed or open groups), type of clients in a group, and duration of group (is it ongoing or does it cease functioning after so many meetings?). As a therapeutic recreation specialist, you are expected to be able to place clients in the most appropriate intervention group based on their needs and abilities. Group leaders need to be enthusiastic and be able to act as a link between individual group members and the group. Not only do therapeutic recreation therapists need to be able to lead specific activities, but they also need to watch members for any potential problems, help with necessary activity adaptations, and engage the patient/client in discussions.

In structuring a group session, there are three important parts: the opening of the session, the body of the session, and the closing of the session. In the opening of the group session, the therapeutic recreation specialist helps the clients relax and get to know each other. Also the CTRS lets the group members know what is going to occur during the session as far as the activity is concerned. The body is the focus of the group's session. Whether it is a game, an arts and crafts project, a leisure awareness activity, or an experiential activity, it is up to the CTRS to be prepared with the activity ready to go. The CTRS needs to keep in mind the outcomes of the activity and then facilitate the activity so the purpose and goals are attained. At the end of the activity it is important to "process the activity." Processing involves talking with the clients about what they think, how they feel, and anything else that relates to the behavior displayed during the activity. Processing is a very important part of the session because it focuses on what just happened and can help the client generalize his/her behavior into other aspects of his/her life. In order to be able to process effectively, the CTRS needs to be able to do the following: focus, redirect, block, link, and summarize (Shank & Coyle, 2002). The CTRS needs to be able to summarize and effectively bring closure to the session. It is the ability to utilize these leadership principles that will assist the therapeutic recreation specialist in providing a truly therapeutic session. No matter how many activities a person knows, if the activities are not led well, the client/patient will not benefit as much as possible.

The therapeutic recreation specialist also needs to know how to safely work with persons who might need assistance in transferring from the bed to a wheelchair or from a wheelchair to a chair and an understanding of sign language might also be useful. Any specific techniques that will assist a client in participating in a group or activity is important for the therapeutic recreation specialist to know (Austin, 2009; Carter & van Andel, 2011; Kunstler & Daly, 2010; Shank & Coyle, 2002).

The content covered in this Background section of Foundational Knowledge is usually taught in what NCTRC refers to as "support courses." It can also be found in introductory recreation/leisure courses and leadership courses both in recreation/leisure and therapeutic recreation.

References Related to Background

Austin, D. R. (2009). *Therapeutic recreation processes and techniques* (6th ed.). Urbana, IL: Sagamore.

Carter, M. J., & van Andel, G. (2011). *Therapeutic recreation: A practical approach* (4th ed.). Prospect Heights, IL: Waveland Press.

Dattilo, J., & Murphy, W. D. (1987). *Behavior modification in therapeutic recreation*. State College, PA: Venture.

Edginton, C. R., Jordan, D. J., DeGraaf, D. G., & Edginton, S. R. (2002). *Leisure and life satisfaction: Foundational perspectives* (3rd ed.). Boston, MA: McGraw Hill.

Feil, N. (1993). *The validation breakthrough*. Baltimore, MD: Health Professions Press.

Getz, D. (2002). Increasing cultural competence in therapeutic recreation. In D. R. Austin, J. Dattilo, & B. P. McCormick (Eds.), *Conceptual foundations in therapeutic recreation* (pp. 151-163). State College, PA: Venture.

Godbey, G. (2003). *Leisure in your life: An exploration*. State College, PA: Venture.

Howard, D., Dieser, R., Yang, H., Pegg, S. & Lammel, J. (2008) A global perspective of therapeutic recreation. In T. Robertson & T. Long (Eds.), *Foundations of therapeutic recreation* (pp. 231-249). Champaign, IL: Human Kinetics.

Iso-Ahola, S. E. (1980). *The social psychology of leisure and recreation*. Dubuque, IA: Wm. C. Brown.

Jordan, D. J. (2001). *Leadership in leisure services: Making a difference*. State College, PA: Venture.

Kunstler, R., & Daly, F. S. (2010). *Therapeutic recreation leadership and programming*. Champaign, IL: Human Kinetics.

Long, T. (2011). Cognitive-behavioral approaches to therapeutic recreation. In N. J. Stumbo & B. Wardlaw (Eds.), *Facilitation of therapeutic recreation services: An evidence-based and best practice approach to techniques and processes* (pp. 289-306). State College, PA: Venture.

Mannell, R. C., & Kleiber, D. (1997). *A social psychology of leisure*. State College, PA: Venture.

Porter, H. R., & Burlingame, J. (2006). *Recreational therapy handbook of practice: ICF-based diagnosis and treatment*. Enumclaw, WA: Idyll Arbor, Inc.

Shank, J., & Coyle, C. (2002). *Therapeutic recreation in health promotion and rehabilitation*. State College, PA: Venture.

B. Diagnostic Groupings

Also a part of Foundational Knowledge is the area *Diagnostic Groupings*. This area ensures that the entry-level professional has an understanding of people with disabilities and the effects of disabling conditions on their lives. The competencies within this area are Cognition and Related Impairments; Anatomy, Physiology and Kinesiology and Related Impairments; Senses and Related Impairments; and Psychology and Related Impairments. These subtopics encompass the disabling conditions that affect the people with whom therapeutic recreation professionals work. In addition to having an understanding of these diagnostic groups, the entry level professional must have an understanding of medical terminology and general pharmacology, its uses and side effects, for specific groups.

1. Cognition and Related Impairments

The first competency is *Cognition and Related Impairments*. Within this subtopic, all disabling conditions that have an impact on a person's cognitive abilities are addressed. This subtopic covers disabilities ranging from learning disabilities to intellectual disabilities. One of the primary populations within this subtopic is persons with developmental disabilities. When developmental disabilities were first mentioned in legislation (the Developmental Disabilities Assistance Bill of Rights Act of 1970) specific types of disabilities (e.g., cerebral palsy, epilepsy) were classified as developmental disabilities. However, when the law was reenacted (the Rehabilitation Comprehensive Services, and Developmental Disabilities Amendments of 1978) a more functional definition was substituted (Carter & van Andel, 2011; Mobily & MacNeil, 2002). A developmental disability is "a severe and chronic disorder involving mental and/or physical impairment that originates before age 22. Such a disorder is likely to persist indefinitely and cause substantial functional limitations in at least three of seven areas of major life activity, including self-care, receptive and expressive language, learning, mobility, self-direction, capacity for independent living, and economic self-sufficiency" (Mobily & MacNeil, 2002, p. 15).

Most people who have an intellectual disability are *developmentally disabled*. However the opposite is not true, many people who are developmentally disabled do not have an intellectual disability. A person who is classified as intellectually disabled has scored significantly (a minimum of two standard deviations) below average on a standardized IQ test. The most commonly used classification system is the one used by the American Psychiatric Association (2000): mild, moderate, severe, and profound. Entry-level professionals need to know what these levels of intellectual disability mean in regards to the functioning of the individual, any special teaching/learning characteristics that are necessary dependent on functioning level, and any activity protocols that have been developed for this population.

Many individuals with *autism* have functional characteristics that enable them to be classified as developmentally disabled. Three out of four individuals diagnosed with autism have an intellectual disability. Autism is considered to be a spectrum disorder because the symptoms and characteristics present themselves in a wide variety of combinations. These disorders are on a continuum from classic autism (severe) to a lesser impairment referred to as Asperger's syndrome. Behavioral symptoms can range from hyperactivity, short attention span, impulsivity, to self-injurious behaviors. An individual can have problems with sensory stimulation (oversensitivity to sound or touch), eating, sleeping, and an absence of emotional reaction (i.e., no reaction to pain) or excessive fear. There may also be a problem with speech (echolalia), poor eye contact, resistance to change, and sustained odd play. Entry-level professionals need to have a basic understanding of the symptoms of autism, its prognosis, and treatment. You also need to have a basic understanding about the unique needs of a person with autism in regard to the environment and leadership techniques.

Also included in Cognition and Related Impairments are persons with *traumatic brain injury* (TBI). Persons with TBI have generally been involved in an accident and may have other complications that involve their physical abilities. It is important to understand the different levels of brain injury; thus, you need to know/understand both the Glasgow Coma Scale and the Rancho Los Amigos Scale of Cognitive Functioning. The Glasgow Scale predicts

degree of recovery and severity of a TBI; while, the Rancho Scale identifies eight levels of cognitive functioning organized into four intervention stages. Also, you need to have a basic understanding of the brain so if an injury occurred in a specific area of the brain, you would generally know what the cognitive effects might be. In addition, you need to be familiar with the treatment of persons with brain injury, the value of therapeutic recreation in treatment, and any specific protocols used with this population. It is also important to be aware of the impact of a brain-injured person on the family (Carter & van Andel, 2011, Mobily & MacNeil, 2002; Porter & Burlingame, 2006).

A group of people who experience effects similar to persons with traumatic brain injury are those who have had a *cardiovascular accident* (CVA) or stroke that is essentially an interruption of the blood-flow to the brain. Strokes may be caused by a cerebral thrombosis, hemorrhage, or embolism. Hemiplegia is a sign of a stroke. Damage to the right side of the brain may cause left hemiplegia, problems with depth perception, visual neglect, problems orienting to the environment and estimating abilities. Damage to the left side of the brain will cause right hemiplegia, and individuals may have problems speaking (aphasia), understanding, reading, writing, and judgment. They may also have problems with new situations. It is important to understand the impact of a CVA on a person, the general protocol used to treat a person who has had a CVA, and, again, the impact on family life (Carter & van Andel, 2011; Mobily & MacNeil, 2002).

Dementia is also considered a cognitive impairment. There are a variety of types of dementia including Alzheimer's Disease, Vascular Dementia, Dementia with Lewy Bodies, Pick's Disease, Parkinson's disease, Alcohol-related dementia, and Wernicke-Korsakoff Syndrome. According to Buettner and Fitzsimmons (2003), there are two sets of symptoms that an entry-level therapeutic recreation specialist needs to be aware of: behavioral symptoms and cognitive symptoms. Although the loss of cognitive skills and memory is disturbing, it is the behavioral symptoms (apathy, physical aggression or nonaggression, verbal nonaggression or aggression, or refusal of care or medication, etc.) that cause the most difficulty for caregivers. Persons with dementia may also experience depression, paranoia, social withdrawal, or suicidal ideation (pp. 11-12). The most common form of dementia is Alzheimer's Disease (AD). There are three stages of AD: Stage One or Mild lasts between two and four years, Stage Two or Moderate lasts from two to seven years, and the Third Stage is Severe and lasts from one to three years. Each stage is distinctive and has its own symptoms. The entry-level therapeutic recreation specialist needs to be aware of and understand the protocols that have been developed for the care of persons with dementia (Buettner & Fitzsimmons, 2003; Carter & van Andel, 2011; Mobily & MacNeil, 2002).

"*Epilepsy* is a chronic brain disorder characterized by recurring attacks of abnormal sensory, motor, and psychological activity" (Tamparo & Lewis, 2000, p. 235). A seizure disorder is a common neurological condition that can be either primary or secondary epilepsy. If a seizure has no identifiable etiology, then it can be classified as "primary." If it happens after an impact to the brain and seizures occur, it would be classified as a "secondary" condition. A "partial" seizure involves only one cerebral hemisphere, while a "generalized" seizure involves both hemispheres. Seizures may also be classified as "simple," no loss of consciousness, or "complex" in which a person loses consciousness (American Psychiatric Association, 2000; Buettner & Fitzsimmons, 2003; Carter & van Andel, 2011; Coyne & Fullerton, 2004; Mobily & MacNeil, 2002, Porter & Burlingame, 2006; Tamparo & Lewis, 2000).

2. Anatomy, physiology, and kinesiology and related impairments

This diagnostic grouping seems to be the largest competency in the Diagnostic Groupings knowledge area. It seems almost any impairment that does not fit under cognitive, sensory, or psychiatric can be found here, thus this category ranges from a total hip replacement to AIDS. These impairments may cause an adjustment in a person's activities for a period of time but may not cause a complete change of lifestyle or they may cause a complete disruption in a person's lifestyle. It is important to understand the treatment of these disorders and the type of adapted equipment that the person may temporarily or permanently require.

Cerebral Palsy (CP) is a developmental disorder that is characterized by problems controlling movement. It is a non-progressive disorder. CP can be classified by limb involvement (quadriplegia, paraplegia, diplegia, hemiplegia, triplegia, or monoplegia) or by exhibited symptoms (spasticity, athetosis, or ataxia). As an entry-level therapeutic recreation specialist, it is important to understand the functional characteristics of the classifications mentioned. As an entry-level therapeutic recreation specialist, one should understand the impact of CP on the individual and his or her needs. Primarily, therapeutic recreation specialists will work with individuals with CP in community settings or camps.

Muscular Dystrophy (MD) is a group of related diseases that affect the musculoskeletal system. Duchenne or childhood muscular dystrophy is the most severe and common form of MD. It affects male children who begin to show symptoms by the age of two or three. This is a progressive disease. By adolescence, most persons who have Duchenne use a wheelchair and by adulthood usually are confined to a bed. Most men with Duchenne die in their early 20s. There are two other types of MD that affect adults: facio-scapulo-humeral and limb-girdle. These types affect both males and females. It is important to understand the effects of MD on the person's leisure, help them make necessary adaptations, and, as the MD progresses, help the person and the families deal with the changes. Again, most therapeutic recreation specialists will work with persons who have MD in a community or camp setting.

Spinal cord injury includes persons who have paraplegia or quadriplegia. Spinal cord injuries are usually acquired through trauma. The level of injury is identified by the initial area of the spinal cord where the lesion occurs. A person whose cord is severed above the second thoracic vertebra (T2) has quadriplegia, and a person who has an injury at or below the second thoracic vertebra has paraplegia. Also the lesion can be labeled complete or incomplete. Thus, it is important for the entry-level therapeutic recreation specialist to understand the effects of the location of the lesion and what it means when a lesion is complete or incomplete on a person's functioning level. The therapeutic recreation specialist is expected to help the individual use his residual skills to regain as much independence as possible and to assist in the treatment of secondary conditions such as depression or adjustment to disability. It is important to understand the treatment protocols for persons with spinal cord injury, the benefits of therapeutic recreation, and equipment adaptations. Community reintegration is an important treatment component for persons who are coping with spinal cord injury.

Multiple Sclerosis (MS) is a disease that impacts the nervous system. It is commonly diagnosed in individuals who are between the ages of 20 and 50. MS causes deterioration of the myelin sheath. There is no set pattern of symptoms, but commonly a person has speech disturbances, balance problems, vertigo, blurred vision, walking difficulties, and tremors. There is a pattern of exacerbation and remission, but there is never a complete recovery to the original functioning level. An entry-level professional must understand the progression of this disorder, its prognosis, and treatment of this condition. It is important to understand the impact of this disorder on a person's life and the adjustments to be made in their lifestyle.

Diseases of the circulatory system are also included under Anatomy, Physiology, and Kinesiology and Related Impairments. A therapeutic recreation specialist may work with persons who are recovering from a myocardial infarction or have specific heart conditions that may impact their treatment. The American Heart Association has established functional ability limitations ranging from Class I (no limitation of physical activity) to Class IV (inability to carry on any physical activity without discomfort). The therapeutic recreation specialist must understand the prognosis of these diseases, restrictions, and assist the person in the development of a healthy lifestyle.

Also within Anatomy, Physiology and Kinesiology and Related Impairments are diseases of the endocrine and metabolic systems. This includes persons learning to cope with *diabetes mellitus*. A person who is diagnosed with diabetes has large amounts of sugar in the blood and urine. Immune-mediated diabetes type 1 usually is diagnosed before age 30. It is usually very difficult to regulate and the person is usually on insulin. Type 2 diabetes is more common and appears in adults older than 40. This form of diabetes can be managed by diet, but some people may require insulin. Entry-level professionals may need to know how to assist people in coping with their diabetes and the impact of exercise on their insulin levels. Often diabetes is a secondary condition and the therapeutic recreation specialist needs to be aware of the impact of this disease on the person with the disability. Society today is seeing an influx of diabetes due to diets high in fats and sugar, and poor exercise habits by a majority of Americans. The therapeutic recreation specialist can have a huge impact on persons with diabetes by encouraging and teaching healthy lifestyles and nutrition.

Infectious diseases are also included within Anatomy, Physiology and Kinesiology and Related Impairments. Entry-level professionals need to have an understanding of a variety of cancers, their prognosis, and treatment. *Cancer* includes a group of more than 100 diseases. A tumor may be benign or malignant. If it is malignant, a tumor is invasive, grows rapidly, and can metastasize through the circulatory or lymph system. Tumors can be graded (1-4) and staged using a TNM system: "T" refers to the size and extent of the primary tumor, "N" refers to the number of area lymph nodes involved, and

"M" refers to any metastasis of the primary tumor. Entry-level therapeutic recreation specialists need to understand the role of a therapeutic recreation specialist in assisting the person in attaining/continuing quality of life. Therapeutic recreation specialists can address the psychosocial impact of cancer.

Autoimmune Deficiency Syndrome (AIDS) is a viral infection associated with the human immuno-deficiency virus (HIV). The virus is usually transmitted through sexual intercourse, but it can be transmitted by blood and blood products. AIDS produces a spectrum of symptoms. It is imperative that entry-level professionals understand the etiology of this disease, necessary precautions, prognosis, and treatment. This disease also requires that the therapeutic recreation specialist be able to help the client/patient cope with an incurable illness and continue a quality of life that is appealing to him or her (Carter & van Andel, 2011; Mobily & MacNeil, 2002; Tamparo & Lewis, 2000).

This section has presented some of the major impairments found in the category of Anatomy, Physiology and Kinesiology and Related Impairments. It is not possible or feasible to adequately cover all the potential physical impairments that an entry-level professional may be expected to understand. The clients/patients you will be working with may be in a variety of rehabilitative stages and it is recommended that you seek more information from textbooks or websites that focus on these disabilities.

3. Senses and Related Impairments

This is the third competency area in *Diagnostic Groupings*. The entry-level professional needs to have an understanding of the person who has *visual impairments* or is blind. A person who is classified legally blind has visual acuity of 20/200 or less in the better eye after correction or to a field of vision that is limited to an angle of 20 degrees or less out of the normal 180-degree field of vision (Carter & van Andel, 2011). The therapeutic recreation specialist primarily works with persons who are blind in the community helping them meet their recreational needs through adaptive equipment, if necessary, and sports. The etiology of the impairment, how people with visual impairments learn best, and what equipment or adapted equipment is necessary to help them enjoy a satisfying leisure lifestyle, are important topics to understand. An understanding of specific leadership techniques is also important (Mobily & MacNeil, 2002).

Hearing impairments are also part of this competency area. Hearing losses are measured by the degree of speech heard per decibel level—the higher the number value, the more significant the loss (Sherril, 2004). Again, knowing the etiology and teaching/learning techniques for persons who have hearing impairments or are deaf is important. The CTRS needs to be aware of the person's residual hearing ability, use of hearing aids, whether the person can hear better in the left or right ear, and the type of communication method preferred by the individual. Also an understanding of deaf culture is important (Mobily & MacNeil, 2002).

Speech impairments, like hearing and visual impairments, may be found in all populations. It is important that you understand the different types of aphasia that may be a residual effect found with some persons who have had a CVA or another type of brain injury. Also many persons who have CP may also have problems with speech. A therapeutic recreation professional needs to demonstrate patience and listening skills when working with these individuals and also understand speech-facilitated technology (Carter & van Andel, 2011; Mobily & MacNeil, 2002; Sherrill, 2004).

4. Psychology and Related Impairments

Another competency in *Diagnostic Groupings* pertains to *Psychology and Related Impairments*. This topic encompasses the impairments of mental health, behavior, and addictions. You are expected to have a basic understanding of the treatment of a range of persons with a variety of psychiatric disorders ranging from severe psychoses to chemical dependencies to eating disorders. It is also a good idea to be familiar with the *DSM IV-TR* and its use.

It is important to have an understanding of the symptoms and treatment of persons with *schizophrenia*. According to the American Psychiatric Association (2000), to be diagnosed with schizophrenia, a person must have two or more of the following characteristics during a one-month period: "delusions, hallucinations, disorganized, grossly disorganized or catatonic behavior, and negative symptoms" (p. 312). It is important to understand that with schizophrenia there is always a change in functioning level. Also, an understanding of medications and their side effects is expected. It is also important to understand the benefits and differences between inpatient treatment and day treatment programs.

Mood disorders are those disorders that have a strong impact on emotions. They include depression and bipolar disorders. A person diagnosed with depression has a serious illness. It is not the typical day-to-day "blues." To be diagnosed with depression, a person must have five or more of the following symptoms during the same two-week period:

depressed mood for most of the day, diminished interest in day-to-day activities, significant weight loss or gain, sleeplessness or sleeping all the time, psychomotor agitation, overall feeling of tiredness, feelings of worthlessness, inability to concentrate, and thoughts of suicide (American Psychiatric Association, 2000, p. 356). A person who is diagnosed with bipolar disorder not only has depression, but his moods will "swing" from the lows of depression to mania. When in a manic mode, the person will have three or more of the following symptoms: inflated self-esteem, seems not to need sleep, very talkative, highly distractible, thoughts seem to be racing, increase in goal-directed activity (feel like they can accomplish anything), and overly involved in activities that have a high possibility for a painful outcome. It is important to understand the symptoms and characteristics of these disorders, the benefits of therapeutic recreation with these populations, and potential treatment protocols. Medications can be used to help people with these impairments, and the therapeutic recreation specialist needs to be aware of the potential side effects of the medication.

Personality disorders are also included within this subtopic. The American Psychiatric Association lists 10 different personality disorders, clustering them together into three different categories based on descriptive similarities. Cluster A consists of paranoid, schizoid, and schizotypal personality disorders. In general, people with these personality disorders often appear odd or eccentric. Cluster B consists of the antisocial, borderline, histrionic, and narcissistic personality disorders, and these people have a commonality of being dramatic, emotional, or erratic. Cluster C consists of avoidant, dependent, and obsessive-compulsive personality disorders. The commonality between these personality disorders is anxiousness or fearfulness (American Psychiatric Association, 2000, pp. 685-686). You should be familiar with the major types and their symptoms, as well as techniques in working with this diagnostic group and any treatment protocols that have been developed.

Eating disorders are also in this diagnostic group. Generally speaking, anorexia nervosa may be diagnosed when a person places himself or herself on a diet and exercise program that eventually causes starvation. An individual who has bulimia nervosa goes through a cycle of overeating and then vomiting or using laxatives (binge-purge). You need to understand the difference between anorexia nervosa and bulimia nervosa, their symptoms, prognosis, and treatment. It is a good idea to understand their functional characteristics, focusing on emotional issues and self-image. Because this disorder is thought to have a direct relationship with the family system, it is important to understand family interactions (American Psychiatric Association, 2000; Carter & van Andel, 2011; Mobily & MacNeil, 2002).

Behavioral impairments are also considered to be a psychological impairment. Within this category are victims and/or perpetrators of violence, abuses, or neglect. Child abuse and neglect have become a nationwide concern. According to Carter and van Andel (2011), "Abuse is an act of commission or inflicting injury or allowing injury to a child, while neglect refers to an act of omission or failure to act on behalf of a child" (p. 384). There are three categories of abuse a therapeutic recreation specialist needs to be aware of: physical abuse, sexual abuse, and emotional abuse. The act of having to watch a parent be abused by the other parent may also be classified as abuse. Most symptoms of abused or neglected children are nonspecific, but the children may be classified as developmentally delayed due to emotional problems, passivity, overly aggressiveness, or other problems. Therapeutic recreation specialists can help these children gain coping skills and self-awareness. Also the children can gain the ability to express their emotions appropriately.

Antisocial behaviors, such as bullying, are also behavioral impairments. Persons who display "bullying" behavior may need help with self-esteem, and the family may need professional assistance. Currently, there is an emphasis on anti-bullying programs however; bullying is not new to our society. Delinquency and criminal behavior can also fall under this subcategory. These individuals usually display patterns of behavior that are not socially acceptable. Most of these individuals can be found in schools or institutions, and prisons (American Psychiatric Association, 2000; Carter & van Andel, 2011; Mobily & MacNeil, 2002).

Addictions also fall within *Psychology Impairments*. Many addictions start out as harmless pastimes, such as gambling or Internet use. Perhaps the most well-known addiction is drug abuse. Polysubstance and alcohol dependence are both included within this subtopic. According to the American Psychiatric Association (2000), 11 classes of substances make up this category: "alcohol; amphetamines; caffeine; cannabis; cocaine; hallucinogens; inhalants; nicotine; opioids; phencyclidine; and sedatives, hypnotics or anxiolytics" (p. 191). Prescribed and over-the-counter medications can also be addictive. Substance abuse occurs when an individual repeatedly uses a substance to the point that it causes serious problems in life, whether it is problems on the job, in role obligations, legal problems, health, etc. Chemical dependency involves developing a reliance on one or a combination of drugs. Addiction is continued use of a drug to the point of a compulsion. At some point, addiction can become so serious that getting and using the drug is the focus of the person's life.

It is a good idea to have an understanding of the different types of drugs found in each category, the symptoms of drug abuse, and the effects of leisure education on the recovery of persons who are dependent on polysubstances and alcohol. It is also a good idea to have an understanding of the treatment protocol for persons who are addicted to polysubstances and/or alcohol. The family system is impacted greatly by persons who are addicted to polysubstances and/or alcohol. The entry-level professional is expected to have an understanding of the impact on the family, co-dependent behavior, and potential family treatment.

People are not just addicted to drugs and alcohol. People can be addicted to gambling, exercise, work, etc. There are people who cannot make it through the day unless they have exercised and have determined how many miles they must run before going to bed. They will ignore their family, work, and other leisure activities until they have gotten the necessary miles in. There are also people who are addicted to work. They do not go anywhere without taking work along on vacation and making sure they are connected to the office through the Internet. In summary, according to Kraus and Shank (1992), "...addiction represents a powerful kind of attraction, for what may initially appear to be a harmless kind of pleasure or personal release, but ultimately totally controls the individual and leads to shattering life consequences" (p. 319). All persons who are addicted could use goal-oriented treatment, leisure education, and an understanding of their behavior and how it affects others, especially the family (American Psychiatric Association, 2000; Carter & van Andel, 2011; Mobily & MacNeil, 2002).

Usually the information covered in Diagnostic Groupings is covered in a therapeutic recreation introductory class or a recreation for special population course. However, some colleges and universities offer special therapeutic recreation courses that cover disabilities only or programming for persons with different disabilities. Much of the information on psychiatric disorders can be found in an *Abnormal Psychology* course.

References Related to Diagnostic Groupings

American Psychiatric Association. (2000). *Diagnostic and statistical manual of mental disorders* (4th ed.). Washington, D.C.: Author.

Buettner L., & Fitzsimmons, S. (2003). *Dementia practice guidelines for recreational therapy: Treatment of disturbing behaviors.* Alexandria, VA: American Therapeutic Recreation Association.

Carter, M. J., & van Andel, G. E. (2011). *Therapeutic recreation: A practical approach* (4th ed.). Prospect Heights, IL: Waveland Press.

Coyne, P., & Fullerton, A. (2004). *Supporting individuals with autism spectrum disorder in recreation.* Champaign, IL: Sagamore.

Mobily, K. E., & MacNeil, R. D. (2002). *Therapeutic recreation and the nature of disabilities.* State College, PA: Venture.

Porter, H. R. & Burlingame, J. (2006). *Recreational therapy handbook of practice: ICF-based diagnosis and treatment.* Enumclaw, WA: Idyll Arbor, Inc.

Sherrill, C. (2004). *Adapted physical activity, recreation and sport: Cross disciplinary and lifespan* (6th ed.). Boston: McGraw Hill.

Tamparo, D. D., & Lewis, M. A. (2000). *Diseases of the human body* (3rd ed.). Philadelphia, PA: F. A. Davis Company.

C. Theories and Concepts

The last section of *Background* pertains to *Theories and Concepts.* These Theories and Concepts are not focused strictly on therapeutic recreation but possibly have been created by other fields and are now commonly used by the therapeutic recreation profession.

1. Normalization, inclusion, and least restrictive environment

The first concepts for this section were used by special education; however, they are now commonly used in therapeutic recreation usually in community recreation or educational settings. A therapeutic recreation specialist must have an understanding of the concepts of *normalization, inclusion,* and *least restrictive environment* and what they mean in terms of programming.

When thinking of *"normalization,"* one must keep in the mind that persons with disabilities have the same needs and desires as persons who do not have disabilities. Thus, in regard to recreation and leisure service, normalization would imply that persons with disabilities should have the same opportunities that anyone without a disability in the community has. Their lives should be as typical as possible: going to school or work, participating in recreation activities, etc., with the same life cycle of activities, expectations, and opportunities (i.e., attending dances, getting married, etc.).

Inclusion refers to a process that "enables an individual to be part of his environment by making choices, being supported in what he does on a daily basis, having friends, and being valued" (Bullock & Mahon, 2001, p. 58). The recreation profession has accepted the idea and now tries to present community activities as inclusive recreation. According to Dattilo (2002), when we embrace inclusion we "recognize we are one, yet we are different, create chances for others to experience freedom to participate, value each person and value diversity, and support participation" (p. 26). Community recreation programs are hiring therapeutic recreation specialists to enable persons with disabilities to participate in any community recreation program. The therapeutic recreation specialist may provide assistance through recommendations of leadership needs, activity, or equipment adaptation, or by providing support to assist everyone in accepting the person with a disability in the program. The therapeutic recreation specialist may not be needed after making the necessary program, equipment, or leadership adjustments.

The term *"least restrictive environment"* is an educational term that was first used in the Education of All Handicapped Children Act of 1975 (PL 94-142) and is part of the replacement Individuals with Disabilities Education Act (IDEA). It refers to placing a child in an environment where he can have the greatest success. Not all children are alike, and that is also true of children with disabilities. According to Devine (2008), "Least restrictive environments are situations in which adaptations would be made only when evidence indicates that a person with a disability needs changes to function" (p. 55). Previously, recreation programs may have created "segregated programming" for children with disabilities thinking this would serve those persons best; however, it is now recognized that children need a program that best fits their needs. For some individuals it may be segregated programming at first and then, when appropriate skills have been developed, move into inclusive programming but, some individuals may always require segregated programming (Bullock & Mahon, 2001; Carter & LeConey, 2004; Dattilo, 2002; Devine, 2008; Kraus & Shank, 1992).

2. Architectural barriers and accessibility of programs

According to Gorham and Brasile (1998), there are three components of accessibility "architectural accessibility, program accessibility, and the skills required to access the resources now available to persons with disabilities" (p. 324). In 1965, the National Commission on Architectural Barriers was established. It recognized guidelines for architectural accessibility that were developed by the American National Standards Institute (ANSI). Currently, recreation facility planners must follow the standards issued by the American Transportation Barriers Compliance Board and those contained in the Uniform Federal Accessibility Standards and the Americans Disabilities Act Accessibility Guidelines (Dattilo, 2002). It is up to the therapeutic recreation specialist to be aware of the standards and to ensure that all recreation areas meet federal, state, and local laws and guidelines.

According to Gorham and Brasile (1998), program accessibility "focuses on the design and implementation of specific activities and other events" (p. 331). How does one provide accessible programming? Just because a facility is accessible does not mean the program is. In addition to the elimination of architectural barriers, the therapeutic recreation specialist must make sure there is appropriate transportation or access to the program, that activities have a range of skill levels and appropriate adaptations, that the fee for the program does not keep people with a limited income from participating, and that the program has been advertised to all people, including people who are deaf and may need interpreters, or people who are blind and may need guides (Bullock & Mahon, 2001; Dattilo, 2002; Gorham & Brasile, 1998; Smith, Austin, & Kennedy, 2001).

3. Societal attitudes and stereotyping

The next competency in Concepts and Theories relates to *societal attitudes and stereotyping*. As an entry-level professional, you need to understand society's attitudes and what you can do to help educate and thus improve some of the more negative or misinformed attitudes. What is an attitude? According to Ajzen (1988), "An attitude is a disposition to respond favorably or unfavorably to an object, person, institution, or event" (p. 4). Attitudes can impact behavior. For years, society focused on individuals' differences, thus

causing people to be unaware of how alike we are. This focus on differences caused fear and negative attitudes. Therapeutic recreation specialists can educate people about how alike we are, thus helping to eliminate negative attitudes. One way we can do this is by using "person-first" language; in other words, focusing on the person rather than the disability i.e., person with a disability, person who uses a wheelchair, etc. Stereotyping people with disabilities is also an issue. When we stereotype, we place everyone into a group and fail to treat them as individuals. When we program, we must keep in mind individual needs and differences (Bedini, 1998; Bullock & Mahon, 2001; Dattilo, 2002; Devine, 2008; Smith, Austin, & Kennedy, 2001).

4. Legislation

Perhaps the greatest impact on people with disabilities has come from the government in the form of *legislation*, which is another competency in Concepts and Theories. There are a variety of pieces of legislation that have impacted people with disabilities in the United States and made access to recreation and therapeutic recreation services mandatory. Presented below are only the "highlights" of the laws that impact therapeutic recreation services.

- PL 93-112—The Rehabilitation Act of 1973
  - Title II trained recreation workers to work with people with disabilities and provided research money for recreation projects.
  - Section 304 made money available for demonstrating how to make recreation activities accessible.
  - Section 502 established the Architectural and Transportation Barriers Compliance Board.
  - Section 504-Nondiscrimination under Federal Grants. This is considered to be landmark legislation for individuals with disabilities and laid the groundwork for the Americans with Disabilities Act. It essentially said that a person with a disability could not be discriminated against in any program supported with federal monies.
- PL95-602—The Rehabilitation Act of 1978
  - Section 311 provided grants for operating and where necessary, removing or constructing facilities to demonstrate methods of making recreational activities accessible.

    ° Section 316 provided money to pay for the initiation of new recreation programs to provide activities to assist individuals with mobility and socialization.

- PL 94-142—The Education of All Handicapped Children Act of 1975
  - Ensured children with disabilities a free and appropriate education.
  - Included recreation as a "related service" defining it as including assessment of recreation and leisure functioning, leisure education, therapeutic recreation, and recreation in school and community agencies.
  - Required parents and teachers to write an Individualized Education Plan for all children with disabilities.
- PL 101-476—Individuals with Disabilities Education Act of 1990 (amendments to The Education of All Handicapped Children Act—changing the name)
  - Required more fully the inclusion of children with autism and traumatic brain injury.
  - Included transition and assistive technology services.
- PL 105-117—Individuals with Disabilities Education Act of 1997 (reauthorization with amendments)
  - Behavioral plans must be developed
  - Transition services need to be included beginning at age 14
- PL 101-336—The Americans with Disabilities Act of 1990
  - Defines person with a disability as an individual who has a physical or mental impairment that substantially limits one or more major life activities, has a record of such an impairment, and is regarded as having such an impairment.
  - Disability has to result in a substantial limitation of one or more major life activities.
  - Four Primary Titles under the ADA
    Title I. Employment
    Title IIA. Government Services
    Title IIB. Public Transit
    Title III. Public Accommodation
    Title IV. Telecommunications

You need to understand the provisions of these important pieces of legislation because they have had, and will continue to have, an impact on the lives of persons with disabilities and therapeutic recreation/recreation services (Austin & Crawford 2001; Bullock & Mahon, 2001; Dattilo, 2002; Kraus & Shank, 1992.)

5. Relevant guidelines and standards

When planning a program, the therapeutic recreation specialist must be aware of federal and state regulatory agencies and their guidelines and standards. As the therapeutic recreation specialist is designing the program, it is important to be aware that legislation such as the ADA has an influence on community recreation programming, since no person can be refused due to a disability. Also programs must be offered in barrier free facilities and be as accessible to all as possible.

Facilities that receive Medicare funding must follow the regulations established by the Centers for Medicare and Medicaid Services (CMS). The Joint Commission (originally called the Joint Commission on Accreditation of Healthcare Organizations or JCAHO) and the Rehabilitation Accreditation Commission (CARF) are agencies that provide accreditation for hospitals and agencies that provides health care services. The Joint Commission sets standards for the following groups of healthcare agencies that might offer therapeutic recreation services: ambulatory care, assisted living, behavioral health care, health care networks, managed behavioral health care, preferred provider organizations, home care, hospitals, and long-term care. In order to become accredited by the Joint Commission, the hospital or healthcare agency must meet established standards. These standards have a strong influence on programming. [www.JointCommission.org]

CARF also establishes standards for hospitals and a variety of healthcare organizations that might offer therapeutic recreation services including: adult day services, assisted living standards, behavioral health, blind rehabilitation, employment and community services, and medical rehabilitation. The standards developed by CARF also address programming issues and the TR specialist must meet those standards. [www.carf.org]

Another major influence on health care is The Health Insurance Portability and Accountability Act (HIPAA). HIPAA went into effect in 2001. Essentially it states that health care personnel cannot release patient information unless given permission by the patient. Confidentiality is stressed. More information on HIPAA can be found at: http://www.hhs.gov/ocr/privacy/. Another federal agency's regulations that the entry level therapeutic recreation specialist needs to be aware of is the Occupational Safety and Health Administration (OSHA). OSHA provides regulations to reduce workplace hazards and dangerous conditions (Kunstler & Daly, 2010; Stumbo & Peterson, 2004).

6. Leisure theories and concepts

As a professional who will teach patients/clients about leisure, the entry-level professional must have an understanding of how people view leisure. The entry-level professional must understand the difference between leisure as time, leisure as activity, leisure as a state of mind, leisure as a symbol of social status, leisure as an anti-utilitarian concept, and leisure as a holistic concept. When working with a client who, when asked, says "leisure is skiing," the therapeutic recreation specialist understands that the client believes that leisure is activity, and so has a starting point for leisure education (Edginton, Jordan, DeGraf & Edginton 2002; Godbey, 2003; Russell, 2001).

7. Social psychology aspects in relation to leisure

Building upon this basic knowledge is an understanding of some basic *social psychology aspects in relation to leisure* that include perceived freedom, intrinsic motivation, and locus of control. Perceived freedom implies that people think they have a choice, and in this instance it is used in relation to leisure. According to most leisure professionals, people do not really have leisure unless they at least believe they have the freedom to choose what they do during their leisure. Intrinsic motivation is another concept used in relation to leisure. People must be motivated from within to have a truly leisure experience; external factors (i.e., other people, money, etc.) cannot be the motivating reason. Locus of control relates to the amount of control a person feels he has over the events that occur in his life. If a person believes that for the most part he controls the outcome of events, he is said to have "internal locus of control." If a person believes that the outcome of events is largely due to luck, the environment, or others, then he is said to have "external locus of control" (Austin 2009; Edginton, Jordan, DeGraaf, & Edginton, 2002; Iso-Ahola, 1980; Mannell & Kleiber, 1997; Neulinger, 1974).

8. Leisure throughout the lifespan

Although there are not specific activities that one must participate in during a specific life stage within his lifespan, one can identify general activities that one might participate in dependent upon his life stage. For example, a single person in his or her 20s is more likely to go backpacking in the mountains alone than a married person in his or her 40s. Understanding a person's life stage will help the entry-level therapist develop a program that will meet patients' interests and needs. Some of the information for this competency may be found under the *Human Growth and Development* competency (Edginton, Jordan, DeGraff, & Edginton, 2002).

9. Leisure lifestyle development

Leisure can influence lifestyle. According to Edginton, Jordan, DeGraff, and Edginton (2002), "The work of a leisure services professional, along with encouraging life satisfaction, should focus on facilitating both social (behavioral) and environmental (physical) conditions that help people achieve optimal lifestyles" (p. 13). Leisure can assist the individual in developing a healthy, satisfying lifestyle. According to Stumbo and Peterson (2009) persons with disabilities may have limited experiences with leisure involvement due to imposed, real, or perceived imitations so it is the responsibility of the therapeutic recreation specialist to assist the person in their leisure lifestyle development.

Most of the material covered in this section of Background Knowledge can be found in Introduction to Recreation/Leisure classes or recreation/leisure programming classes.

References Related to Theories and Concepts

Ajzen, I. (1988). *Attitudes, personality, and behavior.* Chicago, IL: The Dorsey Press.

Austin, D. R. (2009). *Therapeutic recreation processes and techniques* (6th ed.). Urbana, IL: Sagamore.

Bedini, L. (1998). Attitudes toward disability. In F. Brasile, T. K. Skalko & J. Burlingame, *Issues of a dynamic profession* (pp. 287-309). Enumclaw, WA: Idyll Arbor, Inc.

Bullock, C. C., & Mahon, M. J. (2001). *Introduction to recreation services for people with disabilities: A person-centered approach* (2nd ed.). Urbana, IL: Sagamore.

Carter, M. J., & LeConey, S. P. (2004). *Therapeutic recreation in the community: An inclusive approach* (2nd ed.). Urbana, IL: Sagamore.

Dattilo, J. (2002). *Inclusive leisure services: Responding to the rights of people with disabilities* (2nd ed.). State College, PA: Venture.

Devine, M.A. (2008). Person-first philosophy in therapeutic recreation. In T. Robertson, & T. Long (Eds.), *Foundations of therapeutic recreation: Perceptions, philosophies and practices for the 21st century*. (pp. 51-61). Champaign, IL: Human Kinetics.

Edginton, C. R., Jordan, D. J., DeGraaf, D. G., & Edginton, S. R. (2002). *Leisure and life satisfaction: Foundational perspectives* (3rd ed.). Boston, MA: McGraw Hill.

Getz, D. (2002). Increasing cultural competence in therapeutic recreation. In D. R. Austin, J. Dattilo, & B. P. McCormick (Eds.), *Conceptual foundations in therapeutic recreation* (pp. 151-163). State College, PA: Venture.

Godbey, G. (2003). *Leisure in your life: An exploration*. State College, PA: Venture.

Gorham, P., & Brasile, F. (1998). Accessibility: A bridge to a more inclusive community. In F. Brasile, T. K. Skalko, & J. Burlingame (Eds.), *Issues of a dynamic profession* (pp. 287-309). Enumclaw, WA: Idyll Arbor, Inc.

Iso-Ahola, S. E. (1980). *The social psychology of leisure and recreation*. Dubuque, IA: Wm. C. Brown.

Kunstler, R., & Daly, F. S. (2010). *Therapeutic recreation leadership and programming*. Champaign, IL: Human Kinetics.

Mannell, R. C., & Kleiber, D. (1997). *A social psychology of leisure*. State College, PA: Venture.

Mobily, K. D., & Ostiguy, L. J. (2004) *Introduction to therapeutic recreation*. State College, PA: Venture.

Neulinger, J. (1974). *The psychology of leisure*. Springfield, IL: Charles C. Thomas.

Russell, R. V. (2001). *Leadership in recreation* (2nd ed.). Boston, MA: McGraw Hill.

Smith, R., Austin, D., & Kennedy, D. (2001). *Inclusive and special recreation: Opportunities for persons with disabilities* (4th ed.). New York, NY: McGraw-Hill.

Stumbo, N. J., & Peterson, C. A. (2009). *Therapeutic recreation program design: Principles and procedures* (5th ed.). San Francisco, CA: Benjamin Cummings.

II. Practice of Therapeutic Recreation/Recreation Therapy (46.7% of the total test or 42 items)

This content area is one of the most important. It ensures that the therapeutic recreation specialist has a basic understanding of therapeutic recreation from theories to the code of ethics, assessment, documentation and implementation which includes an understanding of activities and how to select the correct one to use and various interventions and facilitation techniques. Most of the questions are derived from content of courses that would be considered the "core" therapeutic recreation courses. These would be assessment and evaluation courses, programming in TR courses, leadership and facilitation courses, etc.

A. Strategies and Guidelines
1. Concepts of Therapeutic Recreation/ Recreation Therapy

An entry-level therapist needs to have a thorough understanding of therapeutic recreation in general and this competency addresses its basic concepts. To understand therapeutic recreation, one must believe in the treatment of the "whole person." This approach to therapeutic recreation fits into the holistic health model. So when a patient is referred to therapeutic recreation due to a stroke, the therapist is concerned not only with the patient's physical and cognitive well-being but also his/her emotional, social, and spiritual well-being. The therapist is concerned with the patient's deficits and strengths, what changes might help her when she goes home, and what adaptive assistance she might need when returning to the community in order to participate in her former activities.

An understanding of the value of the recreative experience is also important for the therapeutic recreation specialist to understand and appreciate. For all people, recreation experiences can provide relaxation, stimulate the mind, allow adventure, enable socialization, etc. Clients need to learn the impact their choice of recreation experiences can have on their quality of life.

According to Kraus and Shank (1992), "special recreation is the provision of programs and opportunities for individuals with disabilities to develop, maintain, and express a self-directed, personally satisfying lifestyle that actively involves leisure" (p. 34). Very often special recreation refers to segregated programming for people with disabilities when inclusive programming is not possible.

The term "inclusive recreation" describes "the full acceptance and integration of person with disabilities into the recreation mainstream. It reflects free and equal access to recreation participation by persons with disabilities" (Austin & Crawford, 2001, p. 11). Because the American with Disabilities Act is now the law of the land, all community recreation programs should be offering inclusive programming.

Using recreation as a treatment modality is different from both special recreation and inclusive recreation. It is recreation used for purposeful interventions using prescribed activities or experiences to bring about a physical, social, emotional, cognitive, or spiritual change in a person. However, this is not to say that it could not be used in a community, school, or health care setting, it is not setting specific but process specific (Austin & Crawford, 2001; Carter & van Andel, 2011; Kraus & Shank, 1992).

2. Models of TR/RT service delivery

The Leisure Ability Model is one of the oldest models and seems to be the most widely accepted and utilized model. It is composed of the following three components: functional intervention, leisure education, and recreation participation. According to Stumbo and Peterson (2009), "The ultimate goal [of the Leisure Ability Model] … is a satisfying leisure lifestyle—the independent functioning of the client in leisure experiences and activities of his or her choice" (p. 33). The therapist assesses the client's need, provides the necessary functional intervention, leisure education, and recreation participation services, and evaluates the degree to which the client met the desired outcomes.

The Health Protection/Health Promotion Model can be seen as having two components: a) helping a patient recover from threats to health (health protection); and b) helping a client achieve optimal health (health promotion) through the use of prescriptive activities, recreation, and leisure. Austin (2009) states that the "mission of therapeutic recreation is to assist persons to move toward an optimal state of health" (p. 9). There are four basic underlying concepts of the health protection/health promotion model. They are: a humanistic perspective, high-level wellness, the stabilization and actualization tendencies, and health.

The Service Delivery Model provides what its author considers the scope of services involved in therapeutic recreation. Its four components include: 1) Diagnosis/Needs Assessment, 2) Treatment/Rehabilitation of a problem or need, 3) Educational Services, and 4) Prevention/Health Promotion activities. "The model is intended to represent a continuum of service delivery—from the more intense, acute-care approach involving diagnosis and treatment found in hospitals or rehabilitation centers to the community-based focus on outpatient, day

treatment, or home health care services that generally emphasize education and health promotion activities" (Carter & van Andel, 2011, p. 23).

The Therapeutic Recreation Outcome Model is an extension of the Service Delivery Model. This model looks at the products (outcomes) of the delivery of therapeutic recreation services. It takes into account changes in functional capacities and health status that, according to the model, will ultimately impact quality of life (Austin, 2009; Carter & van Andel 2011).

3. Practice settings

An entry-level professional needs to understand how therapeutic recreation is practiced in a variety of practice settings, (e.g., community recreation, physical rehabilitation centers, psychiatric hospitals, outpatient clinics, day treatment programs, long-term care facilities, etc.). Much of TR is transitioning from the clinical setting to being more community based. However, it is important to keep in mind that the process of therapeutic recreation—assess, plan, implement, and evaluate—is constant, no matter where therapeutic recreation is being practiced. Therapeutic recreation is a "process" and is not "setting dependent" (Austin & Crawford, 2001; Carter & van Andel, 2011; Williams, 2008).

4. Standards of Practice for the TR/RT profession

Understanding and knowing the *Standards of Practice* is very important for the entry-level professional; it is these standards that must guide practice. These standards were developed by a committee of the American Therapeutic Recreation Association (ATRA). According to Carter and van Andel (2011) standards of practice can be used to "define a profession's scope of service and to measure quality of service delivery" (p. 59). Included in this important publication are a variety of self-assessment tools for program and administration practices. It is recommended that you obtain a copy of the *ATRA Standards of Practice* and understand each specific standard (Carter & van Andel, 2011).

5. Code of Ethics in the TR/RT field

This is an important aspect of being a professional since it guides professional behavior. A code of ethics is essentially a standard of behavior that is expected of all professionals. Codes of ethics are self-regulatory but are developed to govern behavior. A copy of the *Code of Ethics* can be found on the ATRA web site. It is recommended that you obtain a copy and understand the ethical behavior requirements (ATRA, 2000; Carter & van Andel, 2011; Kunstler & Daly, 2010).

References Related to Strategies and Guidelines

American Therapeutic Recreation Association. (2000). *Standards of practice for the practice of therapeutic recreation*. Hattiesburg, MS: Author.

American Therapeutic Recreation Association. (2009). *ATRA code of ethics*. Hattiesburg, MS: Author.

Austin, D. R., & Crawford, M. E. (Eds.). (2001). *Therapeutic recreation: An introduction*. Needham Height, MA: Allyn & Bacon.

Carter, M. J., & van Andel, G.E. (2011). *Therapeutic recreation: A practical approach* (3rd ed.). Prospect Heights, IL: Waveland Press.

Kunstler, R., & Daly, F. S. (2010). *Therapeutic recreation leadership and programming*. Champaign, IL: Human Kinetics.

Smith, R., Austin, D., & Kennedy, D. (2001). *Inclusive and special recreation: Opportunities for persons with disabilities* (4th ed.). New York, NY: McGraw-Hill.

Stumbo, N. J., & Peterson, C. A. (2009). *Therapeutic recreation program design: Principles and procedures* (5th ed.). San Francisco, CA: Benjamin Cummings.

Williams, R. (2008). Places, models, and modalities of practice. In T. Robertson, & T. Long (Eds.), *Foundations of therapeutic recreation* (pp. 63-76). Champaign, IL: Human Kinetics.

B. Assessment

When assessing a patient, the therapeutic recreation specialist must be able to sift through all the information the client may give and determine what is most important, dependent, of course, on the needs of the patient and the type of program (i.e., functional intervention, leisure education, etc.) that the therapeutic recreation department offers. Therapeutic recreation specialists use a variety of assessments and procedures in order to determine the needs of our patients.

1. Current TR/RT/leisure assessment instruments

Although many TR departments use their own agency-specific assessment, there are a variety of published therapeutic recreation/leisure assessments ranging from functional to leisure-based. It is important that as a therapeutic recreation specialist you are familiar with a variety of assessment instruments to determine what is best for the population and setting where you are working. These assessments range from functional assessments (e.g., the Comprehensive Evaluation in Recreation Therapy–Psych (CERT-Psych), the BANDI-RT assessment and the Functional Assessment of Characteristics for Therapeutic Recreation (FACTR) to leisure assessments and checklists (e.g., Leisure Diagnostic Battery (LDB), the Leisure Competence Measure (LCM), and the Leisurescope Plus) (Burlingame & Blaschko, 2010, Porter & Burlingame, 2006).

2. Other Inventories and questionnaires

There are also other inventories and questionnaires an entry-level therapeutic recreation specialist needs to be aware of because they may contribute to the assessment of the patient, dependent on the agency where the therapeutic recreation specialist works; or the therapeutic recreation specialist may be expected to understand the meaning of the results of these assessments for use in programming. These assessments include the Functional Independence Measure (FIM), the American Spinal Injury Association Scale (ASIA), the Rancho Los Amigos Scale of Cognitive Functioning, the Glasgow Coma Scale and the Children's Coma Scale, which are used primarily in rehabilitation units and hospitals. In order to receive Medicare reimbursement, inpatient physical rehabilitation hospitals and units are required to use the Inpatient Rehabilitation Facility-Patient Assessment Instrument (IRF-PAI). The FIM also is imbedded within the IRF-PAI. In many long-term care facilities, professionals may use the Global Deterioration Scale (GDS), the Mini-Mental State Examination, and for Medicare reimbursement they must use the Minimum Data Set for Resident Assessment and Care Screening (MDS). In psychiatric settings, the therapists need to understand the Multiaxial Assessment System, specifically the Global Assessment of Functioning (GAF) (Burlingame & Blaschko, 2010; Shank & Coyle, 2002; Stumbo, 2002).

3. Other sources of assessment

Sometimes it is not possible for the patient to provide all the necessary information for a complete assessment. So, it is important that as an entry-level professional you know to use *other sources of assessment information* such as medical records, educational records, interviews with family and friends, and other members of the treatment team (Austin, 2009; Burlingame & Blaschko, 2010; Carter & van Andel, 2011; Shank & Coyle, 2002; Stumbo, 2002; Stumbo & Peterson, 2009).

4. Criteria for selection and/or development of assessment

In order to *select the most appropriate assessment tool*, you need to have an understanding of reliability, validity, usability, and practicability. According to Stumbo and Peterson (2009), "reliability refers to the estimate of the consistency of measurement" (p. 263). Validity, on the other hand, refers to "the extent to which the assessment meets its intended purpose" (Stumbo, 2002, p. 32). So, does the assessment measure what is necessary to place the patient in the appropriate program and has it been tested on the population in the agency for which it is intended? Usability and practicability involve whether the assessment is "doable" as far as time constraints, ease of use, cost, availability, and staff knowledge and ability (Burlingame & Blaschko, 2010; Stumbo & Peterson, 2009; Stumbo, 2002; Sylvester, Voelkl, & Ellis, 2001).

5. Implementation of Assessment

When *implementing the assessment*, it is important that the therapist completely understand the assessment tool and is able to administer it with ease following the directions that were given to ensure test reliability. The therapeutic recreation specialist needs to easily use strategies of interviews, observations, self-administered questionnaires, and record reviews depending on the information desired. According to Stumbo (2002), there is a seven-step process for the assessment implementation process, including: 1) reviewing the assessment protocol, 2) preparing for assessment, 3) administering assessment to the patient, 4) analyzing or scoring the assessment results, 5) interpreting results for placement into programs, 6) documenting results of assessment, and 7) reassessing the patient as necessary/monitoring progress (Stumbo, 2002; Kunstler & Daly, 2008).

Looking at the competencies listed under assessment procedures, i.e., *observation, interviewing and functional skills testing*, are important knowledge items in this category. The tools of observation, interviewing, and functional skills testing are three of the most important tools an entry-level therapist can have.

6. Behavioral observation related to assessment

Systematic observation is the most frequently used type of observation in the field today. It standardizes the procedures used including identifying the targeted behavior, developing specific recording techniques for the observation of the targeted behavior, and scoring and interpreting the observation. There are different types of recording methods/techniques used in therapeutic recreation including: checklists, rating scales, anecdotal records along with frequency or tally methods, and duration, interval and instantaneous time sampling techniques (Burlingame & Blaschko, 2010; Kunstler & Daly, 2008; Shank & Coyle, 2002; Stumbo, 2002; Stumbo & Peterson, 2009).

7. Interview technique for assessment

The entry-level therapeutic recreation specialist needs to understand and use interview skills, keeping in mind the purpose of assessment interviews, which is to gather information about a client. Most therapeutic recreation specialists use the directive approach to interviewing, which involves a series of questions targeted for a specific end result. Different types of questions can be asked in the interview, ranging from closed-ended questions (i.e., "What is your favorite leisure activity?") to open-ended questions (i.e., "Tell me what you like to do for fun."). A rule of thumb for interview questions is that they should directly relate to the purpose of the interview/assessment. Every interview should have an opening, a body of the interview, and a closing. All therapeutic recreation departments should have developed an interview protocol to use in assessment to ensure everyone is collecting the necessary information in the same way (Austin, 2009; Burlingame & Blaschko, 2010; Kunstler & Daly, 2008; Stumbo, 2002; Stumbo & Peterson, 2009).

8. Functional skills testing for assessment

For functional skills testing, the therapeutic recreation specialist needs to be able to use mechanical measurement tools (i.e., stop-watches, measuring tapes, or other objects) that will provide standardized information (Burlingame & Blaschko, 2010). Functional skills will be addressed further in the social, physical, cognitive, and emotional domains of assessment.

9. Sensory assessment

The sensory domain is a patient's ability to see and hear. Can he/she see to read? Is it functional sight, or is the patient essentially blind? Can the person hear? How much can he or she hear? Is it better to sit to one side of the patient when working with him or her because his or her hearing is better on one side? Also, how is the person in relationship to tactile abilities? Are they tactile defensive?

10. Cognitive assessment

When considering a clients'/patients' cognitive domain it is important to look at his/her functional abilities. Thus, in general, a therapeutic recreation specialist is concerned with a patient's memory, both long and short term, his/her ability to solve problems, and his/her attention span. We are also concerned with our patient's orientation, in other words, is he oriented to person, place, and time? Another big concern is safety awareness. Is the patient aware of danger and can he take care of himself in public? All of these are examples of functional skills that can be assessed in the cognitive domain.

11. Social assessment

The social domain is a unique assessment. Within this domain the therapeutic recreation specialist is concerned with whether patients have good communication/interactive skills. Can they initiate a conversation, maintain a conversation, and respond appropriately to questions? Likewise, are they able to maintain friendships, and can they develop a support network? All of these are examples of functional skills that can be assessed in the social domain.

12. Physical assessment

In the physical domain, the behaviors are more explicit. Therapeutic recreation specialists assess a person's fitness, gross motor, and fine motor skills. They assess a patient's eye-hand coordination and other physical functional skills.

13. Affective assessment

The affective domain may be a little more difficult to assess. When assessing emotional skills, a therapeutic recreation specialist wants to know what the patient's attitude is toward self. How does he or she express emotions? Can he or she express anger appropriately? These are considered functional skills in the affective or emotional domain.

14. Leisure assessment

It is imperative that a therapeutic recreation specialist assess a patient's *leisure functioning*. What leisure barriers does the person have? What are his leisure interests? What are her leisure attitudes? What leisure skills does the person have, and is she well rounded? What does the person know about leisure and is he able to get his leisure needs met? These are some of the areas to be assessed in the leisure domain.

When assessing a patient the therapeutic recreation specialist needs to utilize background information to effectively understand/use some of the information obtained. In other words, one needs some basic understanding about patients (e.g., age, educational level, diagnosis, family, etc.). It is also important to gain an understanding of the patient's past medical history. Multicultural considerations such as the patient's cultural belief system are also important to keep in mind when assessing a patient. The therapeutic recreation specialist needs to "develop cultural self-awareness, use interpreters/translators and involve the family network" (Sylvester, Voelkl, & Ellis, 2001, pp. 138-139) to fully understand the implications of the assessment.

References Related to Assessment

Austin, D. R. (2009). *Therapeutic recreation processes and techniques* (6th. ed.) Urbana, IL: Sagamore.

Austin, D. R., & Crawford, M. E. (2001). *Therapeutic recreation: An introduction.* Needham Heights, MA: Allyn & Bacon.

Burlingame, J., & Blaschko, T. M. (2010). *Assessment tools for recreational therapy* (4th ed.). Ravensdale, WA: Idyll Arbor.

Carter, M. J., & van Andel, G.E. (2011). *Therapeutic recreation: A practical approach* (4th ed.). Prospect Heights, IL: Waveland Press.

Kunstler, R., & Daly, F. S. (2010). *Therapeutic recreation leadership and programming.* Champaign, IL: Human Kinetics.

Porter, H. R., & Burlingame, J. (2006) *Recreational therapy handbook of practice: ICF-Based diagnosis and treatment.* Enumclaw, WA: Idyll Arbor.

Shank, J., & Coyle, C. (2002). *Therapeutic recreation in health promotion and rehabilitation.* State College, PA: Venture.

Stumbo, N. J. (2002). *Client assessment in therapeutic recreation services.* State College, PA: Venture.

Stumbo, N. J., & Peterson, C. A. (2009). *Therapeutic recreation program design: Principles and procedures* (5th ed.). San Francisco: Benjamin Cummings.

Sylvester, C., Voelkl, J. E., & Ellis, G. D. (2001). *Therapeutic recreation programming: Theory and practice.* State College, PA: Venture.

C. Documentation

1. Impact of impairment and/or treatment on the person served

Any impairment that occurs will have an impact on the individual's life and the lives of the people who love and care for that individual. A person cannot assume that if a disability is physical in nature, that only that area of the individual's life will be impacted. Most likely the disability will present the person with secondary conditions, such as a changing social life that can then create other emotional problems. It may also create difficulties in his or her role in the family and in the world of work. When working with a person with a disability, the therapeutic recreation professional needs to keep in mind that the entire family may need assistance in coping and then learning to accept and manage all the new information and skills now necessary (Kraus & Shank, 1992).

2. Interpretation of assessment and record of person served

After administering the assessment, it is important that you *interpret the assessment* correctly. If you have used a published assessment instrument, it is imperative that you interpret the assessment as the manual recommends. Scores need to be interpreted through norm-referenced or criterion-referenced means if they are published assessments. This interpretation of the assessment needs to be documented into the person's record.

3. Documentation of assessment, progress/functional status, discharge/ transition plan of person served

After carefully assessing the patient, it is necessary to enter the assessment information into the medical chart or treatment plan. When documenting the assessment results, the CTRS summarizes the assessment information. It is important to include information about the patient's strengths, weaknesses, the process used to collect the assessment information, and mutually agreed upon treatment goals and interventions. Each problem and strength needs to be written in measurable terminology; diagnostic labels (e.g., depressed) must not be used as a problem statement. The method of documentation used will determine the format of the assessment documentation. If it is narrative, the assessment data can be written in paragraph format; if using Problem-Oriented Medical Records, it may be acceptable to list the information. Also placement of the assessment is dependent on whether the agency uses source-oriented records or problem-oriented records. If source-oriented is used, the assessment information would be entered in the therapeutic recreation section of the chart; if problem-oriented is used, assessment information will be entered in the assessment or data base section of the chart.

After entering assessment information, the CTRS will enter progress notes dependent on the requirements of the agency. After working with a patient, the CTRS must provide periodic updates on the patient's/client's progress toward meeting her goals. The frequency of providing updates on the patient's progress is determined by agency guidelines, accreditation standards, and regulatory agencies.

Different types of record-keeping systems are used for documentation, such as narrative charting, problem-oriented medical records (POMR), and charting by exception (CBE). Narrative charting is used frequently by community-based agencies, adult day-care facilities, and residential settings. Information must be about progress toward goals, but there is no uniform structure or format.

Problem-oriented medical records is a way to organize a chart. There are five components to this kind of medical record keeping: database (initial assessment results, client problem list, initial treatment plan, progress notes using SOAP, SOAPIE or SOAPIER, and a discharge summary). SOAP is a common form of charting progress notes and is primarily used in hospital settings. SOAP is an acronym that stands for Subjective, Objective, Analysis, and Plan. "Subjective" data is a direct quote from a patient; "Objective" is data that is gathered by observation of the patient's actions or behaviors; "Analysis" is the interpretation the CTRS makes from the subjective and objective behavior; and, "Plan" is the plan that is recommended based on the previous information. SOAPIE adds "Intervention"—what specific intervention was used; and "Evaluation" is how the client responded to the intervention. SOAPIER adds "Revision" for changes made in the original treatment plan (Stumbo & Peterson, 2009).

Charting by Exception (CBE) is used in agencies that have clearly detailed clinical pathways or long-term care facilities. When an agency has a clearly detailed clinical pathway that is being followed, the only time it is necessary to chart is when there is a variance or exception from the typical course of recovery. In a long-term care facility, as long as the person is not having any changes in functioning or health, there is no charting on the individual.

These are only three examples of the types of charting used in agencies where therapeutic recreation specialists may work; there are many others. Computers also impact charting, and different software for electronic charting is being developed. Computers are found throughout the facility to ease retrieval of information and the entry of information. Electronic Health Record (EHR) refers to a patient's computerized health record. The EHR allows the team to have easy access to a patient's record and to easily enter assessment data and progress notes (Austin, 2009; Shank & Coyle, 2002; Stumbo & Peterson, 2009).

The World Health Organization (WHO) has two separate but complementary classification systems that a therapeutic recreation specialist may run across. *The International Classification of Diseases* 10th edition (ICD-10) is used to classify disease and is written as a code. A code is given to each disease/disability/disorder that a patient presents. The ICD-10 can be used to compile health statistics and compare reports of disease occurrences between countries. A therapeutic recreation specialist will not be coding but must understand the various codes.

The second classification that will be used by the therapeutic recreation specialist is the *International Classification of Functioning, Disability and Health* (ICF). Rather than focusing on disease, disorder, or disability like the ICD, the ICF focuses on a person's health and functioning. According to Porter and Burlingame (2006) "… the ICF provides codes that health professionals score on a Likert scale to reflect a client's level of impairment with a body structure and function (e.g., moderate impairment of the frontal lobe, severe difficulty with short-term memory) the level of difficulty that a client has with a specific life activity (e.g., mild difficulty carrying out a daily routine), and barriers and facilitators that affect impairment and difficulty (e.g., attitude of family is a moderate facilitator, financial assets are a severe barrier)"(p. 3). The focus on a person's functioning and potential barriers rather than their disease/disorder easily fits into therapeutic recreation. It is recommended that you go to the World Health Organization website [www.who.int/en/] to learn more (Austin, 2009; Porter & Burlingame, 2006).

Discharge planning should begin the day the patient arrives on the unit. Discharge usually occurs when goals have been achieved. The patient needs to be involved with his/her discharge planning in order for discharge to be successful. The following topics need to be included in the discharge plan: major goals or problems, services received by the patient, the patient's response to the intervention or services, received condition of patient when discharged, specific referrals/information or instructions given to the patient or patient's family (Stumbo & Peterson, 2009).

When charting, it is important to know the various charting symbols, any accepted descriptive words, and exactly how to chart. The following is a modified list of charting guidelines:
- Write legibly.
- Always use a black pen, never a pencil.
- Don't tamper with the record, e.g., change the sequence of the notes.
- If an error was made, draw a single line through the error and then date and initial it.
- Do not vent anger or frustration with the family or patient in the chart.
- Document services provided and document if services are refused.
- Document any incidents.
- Sign and date every entry.

Remember, generally speaking, if you are unsure about whether or not to document something, if it is not documented, it did not happen. The entry level therapist also needs to have a good understanding of and ability to use medical terminology (Austin, 2009; Burlingame & Blaschko, 2010; Shank & Coyle, 2002; Stumbo & Peterson, 2009; Sylvester, Voelkl, & Ellis, 2001).

4. Methods of writing measurable goals and behavioral objectives

One of the most important skills a therapeutic recreation specialist needs to have is to be able to write *measurable goals and behavioral objectives*. Based on the client's strengths and weaknesses as determined by the assessment, measurable goals and behavioral objectives are written.

Many people refer to Bloom's Taxonomy as they create their cognitive goals and objectives. Bloom identified a seven level taxonomy starting with knowledge as the lowest level, then comprehension, application, analysis, synthesis, and then evaluation as the highest level. Thus, our clients must know something before they can understand it and they must understand it before they can apply it, etc. Very often Krathwohl Taxonomy is used for the affective domain. "The taxonomy is ordered according to the principle of internalization. Internalization refers to the process whereby a person's affect toward an object passes from a general awareness level to a point where the affect is 'internalized' and consistently guides or controls the person's behavior" (Seels & Glasgow, 1990, p. 28). It is a five level taxonomy starting with receiving, then responding, valuing, organization and the highest level is characterization by value set. Goals flow directly from the needs list and are statements that reflect what the client is going to be able to do at the completion of that aspect of his/her treatment plan.

Based on the goal statement, behavioral objectives will be written. These behavioral objectives are indicators that a goal has been achieved. Objectives (sometimes referred to as outcome measures) must have three components: 1) conditions that state when or where the outcome behavior should occur, 2) an action verb that describes the expected behavior, and 3) criteria that describes how well/often the client must perform the behavior. Thus, based on the above stated goal, an appropriate outcome measure or objective might be: When asked a question by staff the client will respond politely within 30 seconds. The conditions are "when asked a question by staff", the action verb is "will respond," and the criteria is, "politely within 30 seconds." Writing good behavioral objectives/outcomes takes practice. You may find that during your internship, shortcuts were taken by the therapeutic recreation staff. Please understand that those "shortcuts" are not universally accepted (Carter & Van Andel, 2011; Melcher, 1999; Seels & Glasgow, 1990; Shank & Coyle, 2002; Stumbo & Peterson, 2009; Sylvester, Voelkl, & Ellis, 2001).

References Related to Documentation

Austin, D. R. (2009). *Therapeutic recreation processes and techniques* (6th ed.). Urbana, IL: Sagamore.

Burlingame, J., & Blaschko, T. M. (2010). *Assessment tools for recreational therapy* (4th ed.). Ravensdale, WA: Idyll Arbor.

Kraus, R., & Shank, J. (1992). *Therapeutic recreation service: Principles and practices* (4th. ed.). Dubuque, IA: Wm. C. Brown.

Melcher, S. (1999). *Introduction to writing goals and objectives.* State College, PA: Venture.

Seels, B., & Glasgow, Z. (1990). *Exercises in instructional design.* Columbus, OH: Merrill.

Shank, J., & Coyle, C. (2002). *Therapeutic recreation in health promotion and rehabilitation.* State College, PA: Venture.

Stumbo, N. J., & Peterson, C. A. (2009). *Therapeutic recreation program design: Principles and procedures* (5th ed.). San Francisco: Benjamin Cummings.

Sylvester, C., Voelkl, J. E., & Ellis, G. D. (2001). *Therapeutic recreation programming: Theory and practice.* State College, PA: Venture.

D. Implementation
1. Nature and diversity of recreation and leisure activities

In order to be a good therapeutic recreation specialist, one must understand the *nature and diversity of recreation and leisure activities*. Understanding the range of activities from outdoor to board and table games to spectator sports and the breadth of activities within those categories gives a professional a greater depth of knowledge thus be able to provide a more diverse and, perhaps, needed program for clients/patients (Wilhite & Keller, 2000). According to Stumbo (2011a), there are nine factors concerning activity characteristics of which the therapeutic recreation specialist should be aware:

"1. Activities must have a direct relationship to the client goal.
2. Functional intervention activities should focus on the ability of the activity to help the client reach his or her goals, rather than on the activity for activity's sake.
3. Functional intervention and leisure education activities should have very predominant characteristics that are related to the problem, skill, or knowledge being addressed.
4. Activity characteristics are important considerations for the successful implementation of a program.
5. Clients should be able to place an activity in some context in order for them to see it as useful and applicable to their overall rehabilitation or treatment outcomes. A single activity or session is not likely to produce a desired behavioral change.

7. Consider the types of activities in which people will engage when they have the choice.
8. Program to the client's outcomes and priorities.
9. Client involvement in activities should be enjoyable (or at least not drudgery)" (p. 40)

Thus one needs to know a variety of activities that could be used to help clients reach their goals. These activities need to range from board and table games to sports to stress and relaxation activities to social activities. The more activities the therapeutic recreation specialist knows the more diverse and useful the programming can be (Stumbo, 2011a; Wilhite & Keller, 2000).

2. Selection of programs, activities, and interventions to achieve the assessed needs of the person

The *selection of programs, activities, and interventions to achieve the assessed needs of the person served* is another important competency. According to Shank and Coyle (2001), "you will need an understanding of three things: clients, activity-based interventions, and yourself" (p. 157). Stumbo and Peterson (2009) state that there are "three major factors that influence the selection and implementation of intervention activities: activity content and process, client characteristics, and resource factors" (p. 213). There are two ways that a therapeutic recreation specialist can determine appropriate activities either based on client goals or select client goals based on activities. As Stumbo (2011a) states "…nearly every activity can be designed and implemented to meet a client goal, but not every activity can meet every client goal" (p. 47).

When determining programs, activities and interventions, it is useful to review the diagnostic protocol that has been developed for each diagnosis and the program protocol that has been developed for each program. Determining program, activities, and interventions will also depend on the agency philosophy, type of program, space available, resources available, and length of stay and frequency of involvement in the therapeutic recreation program. Clinical practice guidelines are now under development for many diagnostic groups, which will help practice become more standardized. As of mid 2012 only Dementia Practice Guidelines (Buettner & Fitzsimmons, 2003) have been published and widely accepted (Carter &

van Andel, 2011; Shank & Coyle, 2001; Stumbo & Peterson, 2009; Stumbo, 2011a; Sylvester, Voelkl, & Ellis, 2001; Wilhite & Keller, 2000).

3. Activity analysis

As a therapeutic recreation specialist you need to be able to determine which activity would be the most appropriate for a specific program and why one program would be more appropriate for a specific client population than another. An understanding of the purpose and use of *activity analysis* in programming is a necessity. Activity analysis helps the therapeutic recreation specialist examine an activity's physical, social, emotional, and cognitive requirements in order to determine the skills, equipment, and materials necessary to successfully participate in the activity. Thus, activity analysis enables a therapeutic recreation specialist to determine if an activity is appropriate for the patient at the patient's current functioning level or if the activity will assist the patient in reaching his/her goals. In other words, which activity will provide the greatest benefit for the patient? After completing an activity analysis, the activity can be modified if needed, to assist the client/patient in meeting specific goals. Several activity analysis forms have been developed and can be found in the textbooks listed at the end of this section (Austin, 2009; Stumbo & Peterson, 2009; Sylvester, Voelkl, & Ellis, 2001; Wilhite & Keller, 2000).

4. Assistive techniques or adaptive technology needed

When designing the program it is also important to determine any *assistive techniques or adaptive technology needed* by the client in order to become more independent. After understanding the needs of the patient and completing an activity analysis, the therapeutic recreation specialist should be able to make accurate activity modifications and determine necessary assistive techniques and equipment. According to Stumbo and Peterson (2009) there are two conditions that require activity modifications: modification for individual participation and modification to enhance the therapeutic benefit. Assistive devices or adaptive technology can also be utilized and range from simple card holders to adapted fishing poles to specialized wheelchairs to computer based devices (Broach & Dattilo, 2000; Bullock & Mahon, 2001; Kunstler & Daly, 2010).

5. Modalities and intervention techniques

There are many different interventions used in therapeutic recreation programs dependent upon the client population, needs of the client, agency philosophy, and program. The following techniques are not all inclusive. There are many more interventions used in therapeutic recreation.

Leisure skill development is very important to many of the clients that a therapeutic recreation specialist works with and is an important component of leisure education. Leisure skills can range from traditional leisure activities like sports, arts and crafts, mental games and activities, etc. to non-traditional activities like shopping, spectator and audience behavior, pets, etc. (Stumbo, Kim, & Kim, 2011).

Teaching clients *assertiveness skills* is an important intervention skill that a therapeutic recreation specialist needs to understand and be able to teach patients/clients. Assertiveness skills are useful in everyone's life, especially for individuals who have problems expressing their feelings or needs. Our patients need to learn the difference between passive, aggressive, and assertive behavior, and learn to use assertive behavior in their interactions (Austin, 2009; Carter & van Andel, 2012; Hutchins, 2011; Shank & Coyle, 2002).

Stress seems to be a factor in everyone's life these days. Whether it's the stress of a job, the loss of a loved one, or the impact of a disability, the ability to teach clients to understand and *manage stress using relaxation techniques* is a function of the entry-level therapeutic recreation specialist. There are a variety of relaxation techniques that the therapeutic recreation specialist needs to understand and use. A few relaxation techniques include: deep-breathing exercises, progressive relaxation techniques, creative visualization, autogenic training, Tai Chi, and stretching (Austin, 2009; Carter & van Andel, 2011; Dattilo & Wingate, 2011; Meckley, Dattilo & Malley, 2011; Shank & Coyle, 2002; Stumbo, 2011b; Wilhite & Keller, 2000).

Learning to cope is also an important technique to relieve stress. Coping is a deliberate process and not an automatic adaptive behavior. The use of diversional activities can help people learn to cope with stressors. Some people have found that exercise can help an individual reduce tension and cope with stress. People can also learn to rely on social support systems to assist them in their coping skills (Broach &

Richardson, 2011; Shank & Coyle, 2002).

Remotivation is an intervention technique used with older adults in long-term care facilities. It encourages the individual to reestablish contact with the outside world by introducing topics of interest to the individual through group activities that encourage the use of verbal and cognitive skills, especially long-term memory. It usually occurs in a group setting and lasts from 30 minutes to an hour. There is a specific format used with remotivation and includes: 1) a climate of acceptance (introductions and welcome), 2) the bridge to reality (focusing attention on a specific topic by reading a poem, singing a song, etc.), 3) sharing the world we live in (inviting responses to specific questions based on the previously introduced topic), 4) appreciation of the work of the world (focuses on jobs and tasks familiar to them and related to the topic of the day), and 5) a climate of appreciation (summarization of the day's topic and discussion) (Austin, 2009; Carter & van Andel, 2011; Shank & Coyle, 2002; Wilhite & Keller, 2000).

Reality orientation is also an intervention technique used with older adults who are confused, disoriented, and have memory loss. Reality orientation can occur all day through the use of a reality orientation board with basic facts like time, place, day of the week, date, next meal, next holiday, etc. It can also be run as a group with the therapeutic recreation specialists as the facilitators. In a group setting, the groups might review the facts on the board, use various activities to help diminish confusion, and review various aspects of activities of daily living (Austin, 2009; Aybar-Damali, Bell, Conti & McGuire, 2011; Carter & van Andel, 2011; Shank & Coyle, 2002; Wilhite & Keller, 2000).

Cognitive (retraining) rehabilitation is used with people who have had a traumatic brain injury or CVA. It helps the person work on regaining some of the cognitive processes such as memory or sequencing that were injured or impaired. Various activities such as computer games and crafts that would rely on planning skills and decision-making skills are used in cognitive retraining groups. Cognitive retraining also teaches them to use a variety of compensatory strategies. If short-term memory is a problem, the client learns various memory techniques or how to effectively use assistive devices like using a personal data assistant (PDA) to keep track of important information (Austin, 2009; Carter & van Andel, 2011; Shank & Coyle, 2002).

Sensory training/stimulation is another intervention techniques used by therapeutic recreation specialists. It is used to bombard the senses with a variety of stimulants. Sensory stimulation may be used with older adults who are experiencing dementia or children with developmental or neurological deficits. The idea is to use sensory cues to relate to familiar life activities. Any one of the five senses is selected and the individual is expected to relate that sensual experience to the environment or to a memory. For example, a person is given a certain scent to smell and then asked to relate it to something in his past or present, like the scent of vanilla being related to baking (Austin, 2009; Carter & van Andel, 2011; Shank & Coyle, 2002; Sylvester, Voelkl, & Ellis, 2001; Wardlaw & Stumbo, 2011; Wilhite & Keller, 2000).

Validation intervention programs are used primarily with older adults experiencing dementia. It does not try to orient them to reality but to accept their feelings and assist the older adult in resolving unfinished business/conflicts experienced earlier in life. Its techniques are relatively simple, needing only the ability to accept people who are confused or disoriented for where they are right now and to use good listening and communication skills. It allows the older adult to express his feelings, acknowledge his life through reminiscence, and come to terms with his losses (Austin, 2009; Aybar-Damali, Bell, Conti & McGuire, 2011, Carter & van Andel, 2011, Feil, 2002).

Social skills training is used with persons who have psychiatric impairments, mental impairments, traumatic brain injuries, with many other populations. Many people within our society have problems with social interaction skills, understanding of the importance of friendship and how to make friends, the use of manners, etc. Since most recreation and leisure activities take place in a social situation, it is important for therapeutic recreation specialists to teach social skills to their patients/clients. Typically people who do social skills training use techniques such as modeling, role playing, social reinforcement, and homework used to practice learned skills in real-life situations (Austin, 2009; Carter & van Andel, 2011; Shank & Coyle, 2002; Stumbo & Wardlaw, 2011).

Community reintegration is used in almost every setting by therapeutic recreation specialists. According to Carter and van Andel (2011) it "is resuming roles and activities, including independent or interdependent decision-making and productive behaviors, with family and social supporters in natural community settings" (pp. 89-90). Many of the clients who a therapeutic recreation specialist works with have issues returning to the community whether they be social or cognitive or their issues may be dealing with architectural issues that may be new to the clients. Very often community reintegration is a reimbursable program for therapeutic recreation (Wardlaw & Stumbo, 2011).

6. Facilitation techniques and/or approaches
There are many *facilitations skills* that a therapeutic recreation specialist needs to possess in order to effectively assist their clients. The following are not all inclusive and many more facilitation techniques can be found in the books listed at the end of this section.

Behavior management techniques include behavior modification and coping skills. Some people with whom therapeutic recreation specialists work have some behaviors that are problematic. Using behavior modification techniques to help patients/clients learn to manage their own behavior may be necessary. The following will be information on specific concepts of behavior modification. Positive reinforcement is the provision of a reinforcer that will cause the behavior to be repeated. A reinforcer is anything that causes a behavior to be repeated; it can be attention, food, etc. Punishment decreases the occurrence of a negative behavior. Modeling is the demonstration of desired behavior and combined with reinforcement, causes the patient/client to want to repeat the behavior. Time out is the removal of the child or individual from a reinforcer or stimulating event. It is used frequently with children who are having difficulty coping with an overstimulating environment. Token economies are used in some residential settings. Residents receive tokens for specified behaviors; at the end of a day or week those tokens can be redeemed for something of value to the individual (Austin, 2009; Carter & Van Andel, 2011; Dattilo & Murphy, 1987; Wilhite & Keller, 2000).

Counseling techniques are sometimes referred to in the literature as communication skills. Effective communication is important when working with patients/clients. One of the most important skills a therapeutic recreation specialist can have is the ability to listen; active listening lets the patient/client know you heard what was said. Listening skills are both verbal and non-verbal. Attending skills consist of the following non-verbal behaviors: eye contact, posture, and gestures; it also consists of various verbal behaviors, but primarily are the ones that keep the patient/client talking like "uh-huh" or "I see." There are also other verbal behaviors that let the patient/client know you are listening and encourage patients/clients to talk. They consist of: paraphrasing, clarifying, perception checking, probing, reflecting, interpreting, confronting, informing, self-disclosing, and summarizing. If you are not familiar with these counseling techniques, it is recommended that you review and practice them (Austin, 2009; Shank & Coyle, 2002; Sylvester, Voelkl, & Ellis, 2001; Strassle, Witman, Kinney, & Kinney, 2011; Stumbo & Navar, 2011).

Values clarification techniques are used frequently in leisure education programs. Its requirements of choosing, cherishing, and acting on values have benefited persons who are chemically dependent, have psychiatric impairments—both adolescents and adults— or who have mental impairments. According to McKenney and Dattilo (2011), there are three value clarification strategies that are useful in leisure education: the individual clarifying response (help individuals think about what they just said or did), the group discussion (encourage reflection of the patient's ideas within a group setting), and value sheets (raise a value issue within a group). Value clarification groups help a person clarify their own value system (Austin, 2009; Carter & van Andel, 2011; McKenney & Dattilo, 2011).

7. Leisure education

Leisure education is very important in therapeutic recreation as it assists people in regaining a fulfilling leisure lifestyle and may help them understand the importance of leisure in their life, or gain a new leisure skill. Leisure education is an important part of a program because it is an area that is often forgotten when working with patients in a hospital or heath care agency, and is sorely needed when the patient returns home. In the hospital, much of the time is programmed, but at home, it is not. Many people will return home and be unable

to return to work. Leisure education can help patients/clients understand the importance of using leisure wisely, developing a healthy leisure lifestyle, expanding their knowledge of leisure activities, and developing new skills. Patients may have participated in many leisure activities previously, but for one reason or another may not be participating in them now. Leisure education can help them learn how to adapt activities or determine any specialized equipment needed to participate. Leisure education can also help with learning about and utilizing leisure resources. These resources can range from personal resources to community resources or even activity opportunities (Austin, 2009; Bullock & Mahon, 2001; Carter & van Andel, 2011; Dattilo & Williams, 2011; Shank & Coyle, 2002; Stumbo, Kim, & Kim, 2011; Stumbo & Peterson, 2009).

References Related to Implementation

Austin, D. R. (2009). *Therapeutic recreation processes and techniques* (6th ed.). Urbana, IL: Sagamore.

Aybar-Damali, B. Z., Bell, G., Conti, A., & McGuire, F. A. (2011). Reality orientation, validation and reminiscence. In N. J. Stumbo & B. Wardlaw (Eds.), *Facilitation of therapeutic recreation services: An evidence-based and best practice approach to techniques and processes* (pp. 353-363). State College, PA: Venture.

Buettner, L., & Fitzsimmons, S. (2003). *Dementia practice guidelines for recreational therapy: Treatment of disturbing behaviors.* Hattiesburg, MS: American Therapeutic Recreation Association.

Bullock, C. C., & Mahon, M. J. (2001). *Introduction to recreation services for people with disabilities: A person centered approach.* Urbana, IL: Sagamore.

Broach, E., & Dattilo, J. (2011). Assistive technology. In J. Dattilo & A. McKenney (Eds.), *Facilitation techniques in therapeutic recreation* (2nd ed.) (pp. 111-152). State College, PA: Venture.

Broach, E., & Richardson, S. (2011). Therapeutic use of exericse. In J. Dattilo & A. McKenney (Eds.), *Facilitation techniques in therapeutic recreation* (2nd ed.). (pp. 441-480). State College, PA: Venture.

Carter, M. J. & van Andel, G. E. (2011). *Therapeutic recreation: A practical approach* (4th ed.). Long Grove, IL: Waveland Press.

Dattilo, J., & McKenney, A. (2011). *Facilitation techniques in therapeutic recreation* (2nd ed.). State College, PA: Venture.

Dattilo, J., & Murphy, W. D. (1987). *Behavior modification in therapeutic recreation.* State College, PA: Venture.

Dattilo, J., & Williams, R. (2011). Leisure education. In J. Dattilo & A. McKenney (Eds.), *Facilitation techniques in therapeutic recreation* (2nd ed.) (pp. 187 - 216). State College, PA: Venture.

Feil, N. (2002) *The validation break through: Simple techniques for communicating with people with "Alzheimer's–type dementia"* (2nd ed.). Baltimore: Health Profession Press.

Hutchins, D. (2011). Assertiveness training. In N. J. Stumbo & B. Wardlaw (Eds.), *Facilitation of therapeutic recreation services: An evidence-based and best practice approach to techniques and processes* (pp. 237 - 243). State College, PA: Venture.

Kunstler, R., & Daly, F. S. (2010). *Therapeutic recreation leadership and programming.* Champaign, IL: Human Kinetics.

Meckley, T., Dattilo, J., & Malley, S. (2011). Stress management. In J. Dattilo & A. McKenney (Eds.), *Facilitation techniques in therapeutic recreation* (2nd ed.). (pp. 247-277). State College, PA: Venture.

McKenney, A., & Dattilo, J. (2011). Values clarification. In J. Dattilo & A. McKenney (Eds.), *Facilitation techniques in therapeutic recreation* (2nd ed.) (pp. 593-613). State College, PA: Venture.

Shank, J., & Coyle, C. (2002). *Therapeutic recreation in health promotion and rehabilitation.* State College, PA: Venture.

Strassle, C. G., Witman, J. P., Kinney, J. S. & Kinney, W. B. (2011). Counseling theory and practice: Some applications for leisure education. In N. J. Stumbo & B. Wardlaw (Eds.), *Facilitation of therapeutic recreation services: An evidence-based and best practice approach to techniques and processes* (pp. 115 - 124). State College, PA: Venture.

Stumbo, N. J. (2011a.). Selecting programs and activities based on goals and outcomes. In N. J. Stumbo & B. Wardlaw (Eds.), *Facilitation of therapeutic recreation services: An evidence-based and best practice approach to techniques and processes* (pp. 35-52). State College, PA: Venture.

Stumbo, N. J. (2011b.). Stress management. In N. J. Stumbo & B. Wardlaw (Eds.), *Facilitation of therapeutic recreation services: An evidence-based and best practice approach to techniques and processes* (pp. 317 - 334). State College, PA: Venture.

Stumbo, N. J., Kim, J., & Kim, Y. (2011). Leisure education. In N. J. Stumbo & B. Wardlaw (Eds.), *Facilitation of therapeutic recreation services: An evidence-based and best practice approach to techniques and processes* (pp. 13 - 31). State College, PA: Venture.

Stumbo, N. J., & Navar, N. H. (2011). Communication techniques. In N. J. Stumbo & B. Wardlaw (Eds.), *Facilitation of therapeutic recreation services: An evidence-based and best practice approach to techniques and processes* (pp. 67-85). State College, PA: Venture.

Stumbo, N. J., & Peterson, C. A. (2009). *Therapeutic recreation program design: Principles and procedures* (5th ed.). San Francisco: Benjamin Cummings.

Stumbo, N. J., & Wardlaw, B. (2011). Social skills training. In N. J. Stumbo & B. Wardlaw (Eds.), *Facilitation of therapeutic recreation services: An evidence-based and best practice approach to techniques and processes* (pp. 189-218). State College, PA: Venture.

Sylvester, C., Voelkl, J. E., & Ellis, G. D. (2001). *Therapeutic recreation programming: Theory and practice.* State College, PA: Venture.

Wardlaw, B., & Stumbo, N. J. (2011a.) Community reintegration. In N. J. Stumbo & B. Wardlaw (Eds.), *Facilitation of therapeutic recreation services: An evidence-based and best practice approach to techniques and processes* (pp. 367-380). State College, PA: Venture.

Wardlaw, B., & Stumbo, N. J. (2011b.) Sensory stimulation and sensory integration. In N. J. Stumbo & B. Wardlaw (Eds.), *Facilitation of therapeutic recreation services: An evidence-based and best practice approach to techniques and processes* (pp. 339-349). State College, PA: Venture.

Wilhite, B., & Keller, M. J. (2000). *Therapeutic recreation: Cases and exercises* (2nd ed.). State College, PA: Venture.

III. Organization of Therapeutic Recreation/Recreation Therapy Service (13.3% of the total test items or 12 test items)

This knowledge area is to ensure that the entry-level professional has an understanding of the provision of TR services and the administration and management of therapeutic recreation services. Most of the information for this section will come from therapeutic recreation program design and administration courses.

A. TR Service Design

1. **Program design relative to population served.**

An important competency is to have an *understanding of program design relative to population served.* As programs are designed, it is necessary to have a thorough understanding of the diverse needs of the clients to be served. We are accountable for our clients' outcomes thus a program must focus on their needs. In order to do this we much have knowledge and skills in selecting the correct intervention and using the appropriate facilitation skill that will help clients achieve their goals. All populations have different needs; for some we will focus on their cognitive needs, others their social needs, and others a combination. But, you the therapist must have the knowledge and skills to determine what is important for the clients you are serving. Also having the ability to develop and utilize diagnostic and program protocols is very important. According to Carter and van Andel (2011), "Protocols are the cornerstone of evidence-based practices because they describe the 'best practice' or standardization of specific interventions with specific clients" (p. 145).

2. Service delivery systems

One of the competencies covered within the subtopic of Service Delivery Systems is *health care*. The majority of therapeutic recreation services are found in a health care agency, be it a rehabilitation hospital, a community hospital, an outpatient unit, or a pediatric unit, all are found in the health care service delivery system. It is important to understand what makes this service delivery "health care." Is it how the services are offered? The types of services offered? Usually in health care services treatment is prescribed either by the physician or the treatment team. When therapeutic recreation is prescribed, the therapeutic recreation process (assess, plan, implement, and evaluate) becomes activated and specific programs and interventions are determined.

Leisure services are another part of the service delivery system. Usually the client is referred either through self-referral or by another therapeutic recreation specialist as part of the client's discharge plan from health care. Leisure services are usually community based and may be segregated or the client may be participating in inclusive recreation. If the services are segregated, the therapeutic recreation specialist will follow the same therapeutic recreation process to determine the most appropriate program for the client. If the services are inclusive, then the client often can choose what recreation/leisure service they would like to be involved in (Carter & LeConey, 2004; Carter & van Andel, 2011; Kennedy, Austin, & Smith, 2001; Shank & Coyle, 2002).

Education services are another kind of service delivery system. Due to the inclusion of recreation as a related service in the Individuals with Disabilities Education Act, therapeutic recreation specialists can be found in school systems, specifically in special education services. All students eligible for special education services must have an individualized education plan (IEP). The IEP outlines the services that are necessary for the student to achieve his goals and objectives and the IEP can specify therapeutic recreation services. Within the IEP, depending on the age of the child, there may be a section labeled "transition." The Individualized Transition Plan projects "post school" goals and methods to ensure those goals will become reality. This section may specifically address leisure goals and objectives. The therapeutic recreation specialist may assist in the development of the goals and objectives but will certainly provide the necessary programming to meet those goals and objectives, once again utilizing the therapeutic recreation process (Bullock & Mahon, 2001; Lawson, Coyle, & Ashton-Shaeffer, 2001).

3. Understanding of the roles and functions of other health and human service professionals and of interdisciplinary approaches

The therapeutic recreation specialist is expected to understand the roles of treatment team members, such as psychiatric social workers or psychiatrists and their roles in the rehabilitation process. Most therapeutic recreation specialists will co-treat with other professionals on the treatment team and need to understand what each discipline can provide in the treatment process. For example, the physical therapist and the therapeutic recreation specialist may co-treat on a community re-integration program with the physical therapist working on car transfers or walking endurance, while the therapeutic recreation specialist is working on decision making, community resources, or money management skills (Carter & van Andel, 2011).

4. Documentation procedures for program accountability and payment for services

According to Stumbo and Peterson (2009), accurate and complete documentation is necessary in order to 1) assure the delivery of quality services, 2) facilitate communication among staff, 3) provide for professional accountability, 4) comply with administrative requirements and 5) provide data for quality improvement and efficacy research. Therapeutic recreation specialists, like other professionals, are accountable for services rendered and outcomes achieved. Accurate documentation can provide the necessary evidence.

The type of documentation required is set by the agency in which the therapeutic recreation specialist works. Accrediting agencies like the

Joint Commission and CARF have standards that impact documentation. The Centers for Medicare and Medicaid Services (CMS) require documentation to indicate that services are necessary. The CMS requires that the staff complete the *Minimum Data Set for Resident Assessment and Care Screening* (MDS) that includes section F which is "Preferences for Customary Routine and Activities." In the MDS, recreational therapy is defined as a skilled service, must meet the criteria for active treatment, and is included in Section O, Special Procedures and Treatments, along with occupational therapy, physical therapy, speech, respiratory therapy, and psychological services. Based on the information from the MDS the Resident Assessment Protocol Summary (RAPS) may be completed. Third-party payers are interested in documentation because it is from this information they will make decisions about reimbursement. Thus, it is very important that the therapeutic recreation specialist is very clear when writing problems, goals, and interventions used, and responses of the patient to those interventions (Austin, 2009; Shank & Coyle, 2002; Stumbo & Peterson, 2009).

5. Methods for interpretation of progress notes, observations, and assessment results of the person served

It is very important that the therapeutic recreation specialist be able to interpret the medical chart. One needs to understand the doctor's orders, the assessments/notes from other disciplines, and be able to interpret their meaning. Very often it is not necessary for a therapeutic recreation specialist to assess a patient in a certain area if it has already been thoroughly assessed by another discipline. It is necessary for the therapeutic recreation specialist to understand what has been stated by the other discipline and use that information when developing a treatment plan.

References for Therapeutic Recreation Program Design

Austin, D. R. (2009). *Therapeutic recreation processes and techniques* (6th ed.). Urbana, IL: Sagamore.

Bullock, C. C., & Mahon, M. J. (2001). *Introduction to recreation services for people with disabilities: A person-centered approach*. Champaign, IL: Sagamore.

Carter, M. J., & LeConey, S. P. (2004). *Therapeutic recreation in the community: An inclusive approach* (2nd ed.). Urbana, IL: Sagamore.

Carter, M. J., & van Andel, G. E. (2011). *Therapeutic recreation: A practical approach* (3rd ed.). Prospect Heights, IL: Waveland Press.

Kennedy, D. W., Austin, D. R., & Smith, R. W (2001). *Special recreation: Opportunities for people with disabilities* (4th ed.). Dubuque, IA: Wm C. Brown.

Kunstler, R., & Daly, F. S. (2010). *Therapeutic recreation leadership and programming*. Champaign, IL: Human Kinetics.

Lawson, L. M., Coyle, C. P., & Ashton-Shaeffer, C. (2001). *Therapeutic recreation in special education: An IDEA for the future*. Alexandria, VA: American Therapeutic Recreation Association.

Shank, J., & Coyle, C. (2002). *Therapeutic recreation in health promotion and rehabilitation*. State College, PA: Venture.

Stumbo, N. J., & Peterson, C. A. (2009). *Therapeutic recreation program design: Principles and procedures* (5th ed.). San Francisco: Benjamin Cummings.

B. Administrative Tasks
1. Methods for evaluating agency/TR service programs

This competency ensures that the entry-level professional understands a variety of evaluation methods. A therapeutic recreation department must determine what is important, that is, what should be evaluated. Usually it is determined that quality of services delivered, effectiveness of those programs, and the outcomes of those programs are of most interest to the department, the agency, third-party payers, and the receiver of services. According to Kunstler and Daly (2010), "program evaluation is used to determine program effectiveness and to improve services" (p. 242).

So how is evaluation conducted? First, one must differentiate between formative and summative evaluation. When evaluation is formative, it is ongoing and occurs while the program is in progress. Staff can make changes on a daily or weekly basis dependent on what the evaluation data indicates. Summative evaluation is conducted at the end of a program and can be used to compare programs or provide information for the next session of programming. For summative evaluation, the program is completely finished when the data is collected and analyzed. It is also necessary to understand the importance of an evaluation plan and the need to develop specific data-collection instruments. According to Stumbo and Peterson (2009), there are several ways to collect evaluation data: using questionnaires, by observation, or by record documentation (p. 369). The need to establish an administrative schedule for evaluation and determine the program revision process following data collection for the therapeutic recreation program is a task for the therapeutic recreation specialist (Kunstler & Daly, 2011; Riley, 1987; Stumbo & Peterson, 2004; Sylvester, Voelkl, & Ellis, 2001).

2. Methods for quality improvement/ performance improvement

This is the most common method of evaluating therapeutic recreation services and is mandated by external accreditation agencies. Quality improvement is not just one activity but a variety of activities that provide useful data on the quality of care for patients. According to Stumbo and Peterson (2009), a basic approach to "comprehensive service evaluation involves a ... process that focuses on a) seeking out problematic areas that lower quality, b) correcting those problems, and c) evaluating how well those corrections are solving the problems" (p. 376). The therapeutic recreation specialist needs to understand and be able to design an effective evaluation plan, focusing on identifying important aspects of care (i.e., client assessment, treatment plans, specific intervention techniques used, patient safety or risk management, staff training and continuing education, etc.). After identifying the aspects of care on which the evaluation will be focused, the therapeutic recreation specialist identifies how to collect the data, collects the data, analyzes the data, and then makes the identified changes in patient care.

According to Kunstler and Daly (2010), performance improvement focuses on the "quality of the process used in delivering services to the quality of the outcomes produced. Performance improvement is seen as a total management process that should be integrated into the overall operations of the agency on a daily basis" (p. 255). The first portion of performance improvement that is addressed through this competency is *utilization review*. Utilization review refers to looking at how effectively a department uses its resources. Utilization review addresses over-utilization, under-utilization, and inefficiency. This is a program management function that should be in a written plan of operation for a health care agency.

Risk management plans are an important part of all therapeutic recreation services. Every department needs to develop risk management plans for each of their service areas and programs. Essentially, a risk management plan identifies all potential risks that could occur in a facility, with equipment or during a program to an employee, patient, or family member. Then, the therapeutic recreation specialist develops a plan or procedure that will eliminate, reduce, or manage that risk. It involves loss prevention and control, and handling all incidents, claims and other insurance, or litigation-related tasks (Carter & O'Morrow, 2006; Kunstler & Daly, 2010; Stumbo & Peterson, 2004).

The last subtopic under methods for quality improvement is the important area of *outcome monitoring*. In short, "outcomes" are the differences that occur in a person from when they begin treatment or enter the health care facility to when they leave treatment or the health care facility. Of course, it is hoped that these changes will be positive. Currently outcome measurement is being discussed rather than outcome monitoring. The Joint Commission (as cited in McCormick, 2003) has identified three categories of outcome measures: health status (functional well-being of an individual), patient perceptions of care (satisfaction measures of care from patient or family perspective), and clinical performance outcomes (outcomes of processes of care). Therapeutic recreation specialists need to understand outcomes and be able to support positive outcomes as a result of their treatment. This will entail some efficacy research. According to Stumbo and Peterson (2009), "efficacy research is designed specifically to scrutinize how effective programs are or were in attaining client outcomes" (p. 94). This research is usually done to determine the effectiveness of an intervention with a particular diagnosis (Kunstler & Daly, 2010; McCormick, 2003; Stumbo & Peterson, 2009; Sylvester, Voelkl, & Ellis, 2001).

3. Components of an agency or TR/RT service plan of operation

This competency relates to the development of a plan of operation or how the agency or therapeutic recreation services operate. For some organizations, specifically in the community, this will be known as a policy and procedures manual. For most health care organizations, the policy and procedures manual is contained within the Plan of Operation. There are two plans of operation with which the therapeutic recreation specialist should be concerned: 1) the agency's plan of operation, and 2) the therapeutic recreation department's plan of operation.

The agency's plan of operation should adequately include therapeutic recreation services as a component of service. Accreditation surveyors will review thoroughly the overall agency's plan of operation, including services provided by therapeutic recreation specialists. The agency plan of operation should include patient management functions and program management functions, with therapeutic recreation included as appropriate. Examples of patient management functions include client assessment, treatment plans, progress notes, treatment plan reviews, and discharge summaries. Examples of program management functions include a quality improvement process, utilizations reviews, and patient care monitoring procedures. A risk management plan for each area and facility for which the therapeutic recreation specialist is in charge is important to develop. A risk management plan will evaluate the amount of risk that an area, program, or piece of equipment may present and establishes policies and procedures that staff must follow in order to reduce risk.

Every therapeutic recreation department or unit needs to have a written plan of operation. All staff should be familiar with this document and utilize its procedures. The therapeutic recreation department's or unit's plan of operation should have a written philosophy that reflects the philosophy of the agency, have overall goals for the program, and describe the purpose and function of therapeutic recreation within the agency. It also should have information regarding the nature and diversity of activities to be utilized with clients and include information related to both patient management functions and program management functions. Examples of patient management functions within the therapeutic recreation department's plan of operation include the client assessment process, treatment plans, interventions used, discharge planning, etc. Examples of program management functions within the therapeutic recreation plan of operation include staff organization and develop-

ment, quality improvement, utilization review, patient care monitoring, etc. A plan of operation is a requirement for a department and is part of the *ATRA Standards of Practice* (ATRA, 2001; Carter & O'Morrow, 2006; Stumbo & Peterson, 2009).

4. **Personnel, intern, and volunteer supervision and management**

This section focuses on the need for some entry-level therapeutic recreation specialists to be able to supervise a variety of people. Primarily it focuses on the supervision of staff, volunteers, and student interns. The supervision of other therapists is referred to as "clinical supervision." According to Austin (2004), there are two purposes of clinical supervision: 1) to improve clinical practice skills, and 2) to ensure that the therapeutic intents of a program are being provided or met. The three roles a clinical supervisor may perform include teacher, counselor, and consultant. The supervisor and supervisee together establish goals that the supervisee wishes to attain. Based on those goals, the content of the supervision program and a time frame is established. The last step is evaluation. As an entry-level practitioner, you are not expected to provide clinical supervision at this point in your career; but, a quality clinical supervision program will help you grow and expand your ability to deliver quality services. It is important to note that clinical supervision is not a performance evaluation by Human Resources but a process to help someone improve his/her clinical skills.

Volunteers play an important role in many therapeutic recreation departments, and many entry-level practitioners need to be able to supervise them. It is important that when a department determines it has a need for volunteers, that the department establishes a volunteer plan including policies, job descriptions, and a marketing plan with promotional materials for recruitment and retention. It is important that program guidelines be established and that while volunteers may be used for parts of the program, they may not be used for the implementation of an intervention. For example, volunteers may be used to provide animals for an animal-assisted therapy program, but it is the therapeutic recreation specialist who is responsible for the assessment, development of the goals for the program, and the therapeutic use of the animals. Many long-term care facilities use volunteers to "call" *Bingo*™ but if the therapist is using *Bingo*™ as a therapeutic activity, it is up to the therapeutic recreation specialist to determine if the patient's objectives were met and to document the intervention process (Carter & O'Morrow, 2006).

The supervision of interns is another important role of a therapeutic recreation specialist. It is not expected that an entry-level therapeutic recreation specialist would be supervising an intern. However, in preparation for an intern, a department should identify internship goals and objectives, establish policies and procedures, ensure the staff and facility are prepared to accept interns, develop training materials, establish an intern manual, determine selection procedures, and establish a recruitment plan. According to Carter and O'Morrow (2006), there are three major tasks that an intern supervisor needs to provide: 1) communication with and observation of the intern, 2) documentation of intern activities and experiences, and 3) provision of training and education opportunities (Austin, 2006; Carter & O'Morrow, 2006; Kunstler & Daly, 2010).

5. Payment systems

Understanding *payment systems (e.g., managed care, preferred provider option (PPO), private contract, Medicare, Medicaid)* is an important knowledge competency for entry-level practitioners. After years of using the retrospective payment system in health care organizations, managed care systems are now the predominant payment method. Managed care systems have shifted the authority of determining the services the patient needs from the providers of care to the payers for care. Therapeutic recreation specialists are often challenged by the insurance companies regarding the need for their services (Shank & Coyle, 2002). According to Thompson (2001), the prospective payment system (PPS) has the following elements: "1) It is a price-based system; 2) Prices are set in advance; 3) The price is inclusive of all services provided; 4) No additional payment or settlement will occur; and 5) The current year's actual costs do not impact the price established" (p. 252). The PPO was established to contain health care costs, ensure quality, assure Medicare recipients access to care, and it has a beneficiary-centered focus. Medicare is a fed-

eral health insurance program that provides care for people 65 and over, for people with certain disabilities, and people with end-stage renal disease. The program has two parts: Part A provides for hospital care, skilled nursing care, home health care, and hospice services; while Part B provides supplemental medical insurance. It covers physician services, outpatient services, emergency department visits, and medical equipment.

Medicaid is a combined program of state and federal insurance for qualified needy individuals. When finances have been depleted by medical care, Medicaid will pay the difference between income and cost of care (Carter & O'Morrow, 2006; Carter & van Andel, 2011; McCormick, 2002; Shank & Coyle, 2002; Stumbo & Peterson, 2009; Thompson, 2001).

6. Area and facility management

Frequently therapeutic recreation specialists are responsible for *area and facility management*. It is important to understand how the areas and facilities are going to be used. A therapeutic recreation specialist needs to have a good understanding of accessibility standards and requirements for specific recreation areas such as trails or playgrounds or pools. It is important for the therapeutic recreation specialist to develop and continually update a risk management plan for each area and facility. A risk management plan will evaluate the amount of risk that an area or piece of equipment may present and establishes policies and procedures that staff must follow in order to reduce risk (Carter & van Andel, 2011).

7. Budgeting and fiscal responsibility for service delivery

The last competency relates to *budgeting and fiscal responsibility for service delivery*. This competency expects the entry-level professional to have some understanding of fiscal matters. There are a variety of sources from which therapeutic recreation services may receive funding. These revenue sources include tax based appropriations from the federal, state, or local government; grants and contracts; contributions and donations; fees, charges and reimbursement; and a combination of any of the aforementioned sources. It is important for the entry-level therapist to understand the source of program revenue. Most community programs revenue sources are tax-based appropriations and fees for services. Within health care facilities, most consumers are charged directly for services and these charges may be paid by insurance companies or third-party payers. Therapeutic recreation services are considered either ancillary services or routine services. Ancillary services are usually prescribed by a physician to meet a consumer need. Routine services are those provided as a part of basic services and are usually built into the overhead or operating costs.

There are different types of budgets used in therapeutic recreation services. The first kind of budget is a "revenue and expense" or "operating" budget. This type of budget delineates the day-to-day expenses and revenues for a year. A "capital expenditure" budget is related to long range planning and usually spans a three- to five-year period. A "program" budget is focused on meeting goals and objectives or allocating resources based on costs and benefits of specific programs. "Zero-based" budgeting requires that a manager is re-evaluating the programs within their department annually. Every program must be re-justified, and just because a program was funded one year at a certain level does not mean it will be again. A manager using zero-based budgeting is forced to set priorities and justify resources annually. Lastly, a "flexible" budget allows a manager to adjust a budget dependent upon unexpected occurrences like a smaller number of patients or patients who are more severely injured and require different, perhaps more intense, interventions than previously budgeted (Carter & O'Morrow, 2006).

References for Administrative Tasks

American Therapeutic Recreation Association. (2000). *Standards for the practice of therapeutic recreation and self-assessment guide.* Alexandria, VA: Author.

Austin, D. R. (2009). *Therapeutic recreation: Processes and techniques* (6th ed.). Urbana, IL: Sagamore.

Carter, M. J., & O'Morrow, G. S. (2006). *Effective management in therapeutic recreation service.* State College, PA: Venture.

Carter, M. J., & van Andel, G.E.(2011). *Therapeutic recreation: A practical approach* (4th ed.). Prospect Heights, IL: Waveland Press.

Kunstler, R., & Daly, F. S. (2010). *Therapeutic recreation leadership and programming.* Champaign, IL: Human Kinetics.

McCormick, B. P. (2003). Outcomes measurement as a tool for performance improvement. In N. J. Stumbo (Ed.), *Client outcomes in therapeutic recreation services: On competence and outcomes* (pp. 221-231). State College, PA: Venture.

Shank, J., & Coyle, C. (2002). *Therapeutic recreation in health promotion and rehabilitation.* State College, PA: Venture.

Stumbo, N. J. (2003). Outcomes, accountability, and therapeutic recreation. In N. J. Stumbo (Ed.), *Client outcomes in therapeutic recreation services: On competence and outcomes* (pp. 1-24). State College, PA: Venture.

Stumbo, N. J., & Peterson, C. A. (2009). *Therapeutic recreation program design: Principles and procedures* (5th ed.). San Francisco: Benjamin Cummings.

Sylvester, C., Voelkl, J. E., & Ellis, G. D. (2001). *Therapeutic recreation programming: Theory and practice.* State College, PA: Venture.

Thompson, G. T. (2001) Reimbursement: Surviving prospective payment as a recreational therapy practitioner. In N. J. Stumbo (Ed.), *Professional issues in therapeutic recreation: On competence and outcomes* (pp. 249-264). State College, PA: Venture.

IV. Advancement of the Profession (6 test items or 6.7% of total test items)

The content for this knowledge area is usually found in Introduction to Therapeutic Recreation courses, senior seminar courses, or issues courses. Many of these competencies have been covered in previous knowledge areas.

1. **Historical development of therapeutic recreation**

    The use of activities as a therapeutic tool can be traced back to the beginning of civilization. However, its history in the U.S. probably began with the development of some of the specialty schools, institutions, or hospitals for persons with visual impairments, physical disabilities, emotional disorders or developmental disabilities (Carter & van Andel, 2011). Its roots can also be found with the rise of the playground movement, which was used to prevent delinquency. Therapeutic recreation continued its sporadic growth until WWI when the American Red Cross used recreational activities to treat those who sustained various injuries in military combat. The Red Cross continued to employ and train recreation leaders during WWII. In the 1930s the Menninger Clinic, following the psychoanalytic model of treatment of psychiatric disorders, used activities to help clients learn to reduce tension, anxiety, and release aggression appropriately. In the 1950s Beatrice Hill established "Comeback, Inc.," which promoted recreation services in the community for noninstitutionalized people with disabilities and also promoted recreation for persons who were hospitalized or in a special school or nursing home. Also during this time period, Janet Pomeroy founded the San Francisco Recreation Center for the Handicapped. During the 1950s and 1960s, community-based recreation programs for people with disabilities continued to grow. In the 1980s, health care began to go through major changes in order to contain costs. Hospitals needed to be accountable for the quality, appropriateness, and outcome of their services (Carter & van Andel, 2011; Dieser, 2008).

The history of the profession is probably more succinctly written by date as follows:

- 1949—Hospital Recreation Section (HRS) of the American Recreation Society was formed and was comprised of primarily hospital recreation workers from military, veterans, and public institutions who emphasized leisure experiences for hospitalized individuals.

- 1952—The Recreation Therapy Section (RTS) within the Recreation Section of the American Association of Health, Physical Education and Recreation was formed by people primarily with a physical education background who offered recreation and physical education programs in schools that served people with disabilities.

- 1953—The National Association of Recreational Therapists (NART) formed to serve the needs of the people who were recreational therapists in state hospitals or schools serving people with mental illness or intellectual disability.

- 1953—Representatives of each organization formed the Council for the Advancement of Hospital Recreation (CAHR) to address common problems.

- 1956—CAHR established the first voluntary registration plan for hospital recreation.

- 1966—The HRS and NART merged to form the National Therapeutic Recreation Society, a branch of the National Recreation and Park Association. Thus, NTRS also became responsible for administration of the voluntary registration plan.

- 1981—The NTRS Registration Board separated from NTRS/NRPA and became an independent certifying body for the therapeutic recreation profession: the National Council for Therapeutic Recreation Certification (NCTRC).

- 1984—The American Therapeutic Recreation Association was established.

- 1998—Alliance for Therapeutic Recreation was formed which enabled the Board members of NTRS and ATRA to communicate and work together on specific issues.

- 2010—NRPA dissolved all branches and NTRS was replaced with the Therapeutic Recreation/Inclusion network. NTRS Board voted to remove the name Therapeutic Recreation from the network and it is now the Inclusion Network (personal communication, B. Wolfe, February 2012).

Because the above outline does not go into depth, the reader is encouraged to read entry-level texts to gain an understanding of how and why these organizations came into existence (Carter, & van Andel, 2011; Dieser, 2008; Kraus & Shank, 1992).

2. Accreditation standards and regulations

This subtopic ensures that the entry-level professional has a working knowledge of the accrediting bodies and their regulations. The Centers for Medicare and Medicaid Services (CMS) is responsible for establishing regulations for both Medicare and Medicaid. CMS was formerly the Health Care Financing Administration. It is important to keep track of the regulations established by CMS if you have patients who are receiving funding from Medicare or Medicaid. Although not an accrediting body, CMS is usually discussed with the Joint Commission and CARF, due to its regulatory nature. The Joint Commission accredits a variety of hospitals and facilities. CARF also mandates standards that relate directly to the provision of therapeutic recreation services (Carter & van Andel, 2011; Shank & Coyle, 2002; Stumbo & Peterson, 2009).

The Council on Accreditation for Parks, Recreation, Tourism and Related Professions (COAPRT) is responsible for the revision and administration of the standards for the accreditation of recreation education programs in colleges and universities. It is also responsible for the creation and administration of the standards for a therapeutic recreation option. The Council for the Accreditation of Recreation Therapy Education (CARTE) has established standards for recreation therapy education. This accreditation program is part of the Commission on Accreditation for Allied Health Education Programs (CAAHEP). CARTE is a new accreditation program with the first education program being accredited in Fall 2011.

3. Professionalism: Professional behavior and professional development

This competency suggests that the entry-level therapist knows what a professional is, what the qualities of a professional are, and what it means to be professional. Austin (2002) suggests there are nine qualities that help define *professionalism*. The first is an appropriate educational background, meaning that you should have received a degree in therapeutic recreation or recreation with an emphasis in therapeutic recreation with the appropriate quantity and quality of coursework that prepares you to work in the field. Following graduation, you should feel like you are ready to practice. Second, you should have a professional organization as your major reference. ATRA is our professional organization. Many states also have Chapters of the ATRA. These chapters can provide you with a local contact and resources. You should attend conferences and read literature from that organization to keep you up-to-date on trends and issues within the field. The third quality a professional has is the individual beliefs in autonomy and self-regulation. The person follows a specific code of ethics and standard of practice. They believe they can make their own professional judgments. Fourth, you should believe in the value of your profession. Do you believe that therapeutic recreation is important, and do you behave in a way that demonstrates that belief by advocating for the profession? The fifth quality relates to having a calling to the profession. Do you believe that this is something you just have to do; you truly believe that therapeutic recreation is something that you have been drawn to and you must work in the field to be satisfied? The fifth quality is contributing to the body of knowledge. Whether it is participating in research, writing an article for a newsletter or a book, a professional makes contributions to the body of knowledge. Providing professional and community service is the sixth quality. A professional takes an active role in a professional organization, whether it is at the local or national level and also works to improve services in the community for people with disabilities. The seventh quality states that a professional will continue to grow and learn by attending conferences or reading professional literature. And the last quality relates to theory-based practice. Every professional should follow the therapeutic recreation process, accept and follow a practice model, and continue to read and incorporate techniques that have been researched and accepted as an appropriate intervention technique (Austin, 2002; Carter & van Andel, 2011; Kraus & Shank, 1992; Kunstler & Daly, 2010).

When a person demonstrates professional behavior, he or she is professionally involved. This involvement may include attendance or presentations at professional conferences, providing leadership in professional organizations, advocating for the profession, and reading and implementing research found in professional journals (Lord, 2006).

4. Requirements for TR/RT credentialing

There are two paths to certification; the first and most common path is the academic path. To qualify for the academic path, an individual must have a major in therapeutic recreation or a major in recreation with an option in therapeutic recreation. The major in therapeutic recreation must contain a minimum of 18 semester hours (for this section all hours are calculated to semester hours—for quarter-hours please go to the NCTRC website) of therapeutic recreation and general recreation content coursework with no less than 15 semester hours in therapeutic recreation content. A minimum of five courses in therapeutic recreation is required and each course must be for three credit hours. Effective January 2013 there will be content specific therapeutic recreation coursework required. It will include assessment, TR process, and advancement of the profession. There must be support coursework totaling 18 semester hours, including three hours of course work in anatomy and physiology, three hours in abnormal psychology, and three hours in human growth and development across the lifespan. The remaining hours must be taken in approved human service areas. Also, the applicant must complete a minimum of 560 hours, 14 consecutive weeks of field placement (internship) in an agency that uses the TR process and be supervised by a certified therapeutic recreation specialist. Lastly, the university supervisor must also be a CTRS (retrieved from www.NCTRC.org, July 28, 2012).

The second path to certification is through the equivalency path. There are two (2) equivalency paths to certification. Like the academic path, all individuals must take 18 semester hours in therapeutic recreation and general recreation course work with 15 of those hours being in therapeutic recreation. The supportive coursework requirements are different dependent upon whether the person takes equivalency path A or B. Under the equivalency path, full-time paid work experience can be substituted for the field placement requirement. Please visit the NCTRC website for the equivalency standards.

After submitting college transcripts to NCTRC and the application to sit for the exam, the applicant will be notified whether he is eligible to sit for the exam. If there is an error or the individual is not eligible, the applicant may appeal. If the applicant meets the standards, he will be notified that he may sit for the exam.

Annual renewal and recertification are two important processes a therapeutic recreation specialist must be aware of. The certification cycle is five years in length. Each year of that cycle the certified individual must submit an annual maintenance application and fee. There are two different options from which a certified person can choose in order to become recertified. The first option consists of a combination of professional experience and continuing education; the second option is simply retaking and passing the national exam. If a person is interested it is possible to obtain a "specialty certification" for their recertification in one of the following areas: physical medicine/rehabilitation, geriatrics, developmental disabilities, behavioral health, or community inclusion services. Please visit the NCTRC website for information regarding the requirements for recertification and what opportunities are available for continuing education.

Licensure is the most restrictive form of credentialing. It requires a governmental agency to enact legislation that defines professional practice. At this time (July 2012) only four states have licensure (Utah, North Carolina, New Hampshire, and Oklahoma) while several other states are working to enact TR/RT licensure in their state. (NCTRC, 2012; Carter & van Andel, 2011; Kunstler & Daly, 2010; Lord, 2008).

5. Advocacy for persons served

A therapeutic recreation specialist is expected to provide *advocacy*. To advocate means to recommend or plead for a specific cause or policy and speak on behalf of another. Very often, it is up to the therapeutic recreation specialist to advocate for recreation services for specific clients/patients especially when they return to the community. They may also advocate for clients'/patients' specific needs in treatment team meetings to ensure that a client/patient receives the treatment or equipment that he or she requires. Another kind of advocacy that a professional is expected to do is to advocate for their profession. Whether it is advocating for legislative recognition or recognition by the treatment team regarding the importance of therapeutic recreation, the professional must be willing to speak up in support of his or her profession (Bullock & Mahon, 2001; Carter & LeConey, 2004; Dattilo, 2002).

6. Legislation and regulations pertaining to therapeutic recreation

This topic has been well covered in Foundational Knowledge, Theories and Concepts. However, one initiative was not previously mentioned that should involve therapeutic recreation specialists. That initiative is *Healthy People 2020*. One of the focus areas speaks directly to Disability and Health. The *Healthy People 2020* initiative is building on *Healthy People 2010* by providing "A renewed focus on identifying, measuring, tracking, and reducing health disparities through a determinants of health approach" (retrieved from Healthypeople.gov, July 2012). Therapeutic recreation specialists need to be aware of this initiative and work within their community to support and assist in the improvement of the health and well-being of persons with disabilities.

7. Professional standards and ethical guide lines pertaining to the TR/RT profession

It is important that entry-level professionals be aware of the *professional standards and ethical guidelines* that pertain to therapeutic recreation. The professional needs to understand and utilize the ATRA *Standards of Practice*. The ATRA *Code of Ethics* and those guidelines should also be understood. Both the *Codes of Ethics* and the *Standards of Practice* were reviewed in the knowledge area of Practice of Therapeutic

Recreation/Recreation Therapy, Strategies and Guidelines (Kunstler & Daly, 2010).

The National Council for Therapeutic Recreation Certification (NCTRC) is responsible for standards for the certification of therapeutic recreation personnel. It is also responsible for placing sanctions on any individual who has violated any NCTRC Certification Standards or any other NCTRC standard, policy, or procedure.

8. Public relations, promotion and marketing of the TR/RT profession

If the profession is to continue, it is very important that every professional be involved in *public relations, promotion, and marketing* of the therapeutic recreation profession. This competency is instrumental in ensuring that therapeutic recreation has a part in the health care arena. Very often therapeutic recreation services can be marketed using the "value added" approach. Thus, the addition of or continued use of therapeutic recreation services will improve quality of care for a health care agency. It is important to be able to promote and market therapeutic recreation at the local, state, and national level to legislators, health care providers, and third-party payers. It is also important to be able to market therapeutic recreation to other health care providers especially physicians and members of the treatment team (Carter & van Andel, 2011; Carter & O'Morrow, 2006).

9. Methods, resources and references for maintaining and upgrading professional competencies

This competency expects the entry-level professional to understand the importance of continuing education. In order to maintain certification, the therapeutic recreation specialist must demonstrate her willingness to participate in continuing education opportunities. NCTRC recognizes a variety of methods that a person can utilize in order to receive continuing education units (CEUs), each method the person chooses must relate to one of the NCTRC Job Analysis Knowledge areas. These methods include: taking courses for academic credit; attending therapeutic recreation continuing education programs at conferences and workshops, writing publications; making presentations at seminars and conferences or presenting guest lectures in courses; and making poster presentations.

ATRA has developed a series of methods for continuing education which can be found online. It acknowledges that continuing education is important to all professionals, and formal education through colleges and universities is not the only way to attain educational competencies. It provides a variety of methods to receive CEUs including conferences, webinars, the *ATRA Newsletter*, and ATRA's research journal, the *Annual on Therapeutic Recreation*.

10. Professional associations and organizations

The entry-level professional needs to be aware of and preferably be a member of the ATRA. It is a good idea to understand under what circumstances it was formed and the purposes/goals of the organization. There are state and local organizations that also play a role in the profession. The entry-level professional needs to understand the purposes of these important associations and become an active member. It is vital to understand that NCTRC is not a professional organization but a certifying body, thus differing from ATRA in goals, purpose, activities, and membership. The history of these organizations can be found in competency one of this Knowledge area. More information on the services our professional organization and our credentialing organization provide can be found on their web sites.

11. Partnership between higher education and direct service providers to provide internships and to produce, understand and interpret research for advancement of the TR/RT profession

As the saying goes, "It takes a village to raise a child," and it certainly takes a community of people collaborating to make a strong profession. The profession expects collaboration between practitioners and educators in internships, research, presentations at conferences, and the authoring of articles and books. Together these professionals can develop and promote a healthy and strong profession. When thinking about internships, practitioners expect educators to provide them with students who have an understanding of therapeutic recreation, understand the population they are about to work with, have leadership and programming skills, and an understanding of a variety of interventions and facilitation techniques. Educators expect practitioners to establish a solid internship program that will take the student to the next level that of entry-level practitioner. It is in the internship that students will put into practice much of what they have learned in the classroom.

Practitioners and educators also depend on each other to do quality research. Both efficacy and effectiveness research can be done as a partnership. According to Stumbo and Peterson (2009) efficacy research questions how an intervention performs under ideal or more controlled circumstances; effectiveness research evaluates interventions as they are actually practiced with clients. Program evaluation is a form of effectiveness research. Very often it is educators who have the research skills and the practitioners who have the clients and programs, thus making each valuable to the other (Stumbo & Peterson, 2009).

12. The value of continuing education and in-service training for the advancement of the TR/RT profession

Very often entry-level practitioners can only see that they need continuing education and in-service training to maintain their certification. However, it is through continuing education and in-service training that we learn more about our clients, gain new intervention skills, and ultimately improve our practice. We also learn to network with other professionals who also can impact on our knowledge and skills.

References Related to Advancement of the Profession

American Therapeutic Recreation Association. (2009). *Code of ethics.* Alexandria, VA: Author.

American Therapeutic Recreation Association. (1998). *Finding the path: Ethics in action.* Hattiesburg, MS: Author.

American Therapeutic Recreation Association. (2000). *Standards for the practice of therapeutic recreation and self assessment guide* (2nd ed.). Alexandria, VA: Author.

Austin, D. R. (2002). Professionalism. In D. R. Austin, J. Dattilo, & B. P. McCormick (Eds.), *Conceptual foundations for therapeutic recreation* (pp. 265-271). State College, PA: Venture.

Austin, D. R. (2009). *Therapeutic recreation processes and techniques* (6th ed.). Urbana, IL: Sagamore.

Bullock, C. C., & Mahon, M. J. (2001). *Introduction to recreation services for people with disabilities: A person-centered approach.* Urbana, IL: Sagamore.

Carter, M. J., & LeConey, S. P. (2004). *Therapeutic recreation in the community: An inclusive approach* (2nd ed.). Urbana, IL: Sagamore.

Carter, M. J., & van Andel, G.E. (2010). *Therapeutic recreation: A practical approach* (4th ed.). Prospect Heights, IL: Waveland Press.

Dattilo, J. (2002). *Inclusive leisure services: Responding to the rights of people with disabilities* (2nd ed.). State College, PA: Venture.

Dieser, R. (2008). History of therapeutic recreation. In T. Robertson & T. Long (Eds.), *Foundations of therapeutic recreation* (pp. 13 - 28). Champaign, IL: Human Kinetics.

Kraus, R., & Shank, J. (1992). *Therapeutic recreation service: Principles and practices* (4th ed.). Dubuque, IA: Wm. C. Brown.

Kunstler, R., & Daly, F. S. (2010). *Therapeutic recreation leadership and programming.* Champaign, IL: Human Kinetics.

Lord, M. A. (2008). Professional opportunities in therapeutic recreation. In T. Robertson & T. Long (Eds.), *Foundations of therapeutic recreation* (pp. 31–50). Champaign, IL: Human Kinetics.

National Council for Therapeutic Recreation Certification. (2012). *Information for new candidates.* New City, NY: Author.

Carter, M. J., & O'Morrow, J. S., (2006). *Effective management in therapeutic recreation services* (2nd. ed). State College, PA: Venture.

Shank, J., & Coyle, C. (2002). *Therapeutic recreation in health promotion and rehabilitation.* State College, PA: Venture.

Stumbo, N. J., & Peterson, C. A. (2009). *Therapeutic recreation program design: Principles and procedures* (5th ed.). San Francisco: Benjamin Cummings.

Bibliography

Ajzen, I. (1988). *Attitudes, personality and behavior.* Chicago, IL: The Dorsey Press

American Psychiatric Association. (2002). *Diagnostic and statistical manual of mental disorders—text revision* (4th ed.). Washington, D.C.: Author.

American Therapeutic Recreation Association. (2009). *Code of ethics.* Alexandria, VA: Author.

American Therapeutic Recreation Association. (1998). *Finding the path: Ethics in action.* Hattiesburg, MS: Author.

American Therapeutic Recreation Association. (2000). *Standards for the practice of therapeutic recreation and self-assessment guide* (2nd ed.). Alexandria, VA: Author.

Austin, D. R. (2009). *Therapeutic recreation processes and techniques* (6th ed.). Urbana, IL: Sagamore.

Austin, D. R., Dattilo, J., & McCormick B. P. (Eds.). (2002). *Conceptual foundations in therapeutic recreation.* State College, PA: Venture.

Austin, D. R., & Crawford, M. E. (Eds.). (2001). *Therapeutic recreation: An introduction.* Needham Heights, MA: Allyn & Bacon.

Brasile, F., Skalko, T. K., & Burlingame, J. (1998). *Issues of a dynamic profession.* Enumclaw, WA: Idyll Arbor, Inc.

Buettner L., & Fitzsimmons, S. (2003). *Dementia practice guideline for recreational therapy: Treatment of disturbing behaviors.* Alexandria, VA: American Therapeutic Recreation Association.

Bullock, C. C., & Mahon, M. J. (2001). *Introduction to recreation services for people with disabilities: A person-centered approach.* Urbana, IL: Sagamore.

Burlingame, J., & Blaschko, T. M. (2010). *Assessment tools for recreational therapy* (4th ed.). Ravensdale, WA: Idyll Arbor.

Carter, M. J., & LeConey, S. P. (2004). *Therapeutic recreation in the community: An inclusive approach* (2nd ed.). Urbana, IL: Sagamore.

Carter, M. J., & van Andel, G.E. (2010). *Therapeutic recreation: A practical approach* (4th ed.). Prospect Heights, IL: Waveland Press

Carter, M. J., & O'Morrow, G. S. (2006). *Effective management in therapeutic recreation service.* (2nd ed.). State College, PA: Venture.

Coyne, P., & Fullerton, A. (2004). *Supporting individuals with autism spectrum disorder in recreation.* Champaign, IL: Sagamore.

Dattilo, J. (2002). *Inclusive leisure services: Responding to the rights of people with disabilities* (2nd ed.). State College, PA: Venture.

Dattilo, J., & McKenney, A. (Eds.). (2011). *Facilitation techniques in therapeutic recreation* (2nd. ed.). State College, PA: Venture.

Dattilo, J., & Murphy, W. D. (1987). *Behavior modification in therapeutic recreation.* State College, PA: Venture.

Edginton, C. R., Jordan, D. J., DeGraaf, D. G., & Edginton, S. R. (2002). *Leisure and life satisfaction: Foundational perspectives* (3rd ed.). Boston, MA: McGraw Hill.

Feil, N. (1993). *The validation breakthrough.* Baltimore, MD: Health Professions Press.

Godbey, G. (2003). *Leisure in your life: An exploration.* State College, PA: Venture.

Iso-Ahola, S. E. (1980). *The social psychology of leisure and recreation.* Dubuque, IA: Wm. C. Brown.

Jordan, D. J. (2001). *Leadership in leisure services: Making a difference.* State College, PA: Venture.

Kraus, R., & Shank, J. (1992). *Therapeutic recreation service: Principles and practices* (4th ed.). Dubuque, IA: Wm. C. Brown.

Kunstler, R., & Daly, F. S. (2010). *Therapeutic recreation leadership and programming.* Champaign, IL: Human Kinetics.

Mannell, R. C., & Kleiber, D. (1997). *A social psychology of leisure.* State College, PA: Venture.

Melcher, S. (1999). *Introduction to writing goals and objectives.* State College, PA: Venture.

Mobily, K. E., & MacNeil, R. D. (2002). *Therapeutic recreation and the nature of disabilities.* State College, PA: Venture.

Mobily, K. E., & Ostiguy, L. J. (2004). *Introduction to therapeutic recreation: U.S. and Canadian perspectives.* State College, PA: Venture.

National Council for Therapeutic Recreation Certification. (2012). *Information for new applicants.* New City, NY: Author.

Neulinger, J. (1974). *The psychology of leisure.* Springfield, IL: Charles C. Thomas.

Porter, H., & Burlingame, J. (2006). *Recreational therapy handbook of practice: ICF-based diagnosis and treatment.* Enumclaw, WA: Idyll Arbor.

Robertson, T., & Long, T. (Eds.). (2008). *Foundations of therapeutic recreation.* Champaign, IL: Human Kinetics.

Russell, R. V. (2001). *Leadership in recreation* (2nd ed.). Boston, MA: McGraw Hill.

Seels, B., & Glasgow, Z. (1990). *Exercises in instructional design.* Columbus, OH: Merrill Publishing Company.

Shank, J., & Coyle, C. (2002). *Therapeutic recreation in health promotion and rehabilitation.* State College, PA: Venture.

Sherrill, C. (2004). *Adapted physical activity, recreation and sport: Cross disciplinary and lifespan* (6th ed.). Boston: McGraw Hill.

Smith, R., Austin, D., & Kennedy, D. (2001). *Inclusive and special recreation: Opportunities for persons with disabilities* (4th ed.). New York, NY: McGraw-Hill

Stumbo, N. J. (2002). *Client assessment in therapeutic recreation services.* State College, PA: Venture.

Stumbo, N. J. (Ed.). (2003). *Client outcomes in therapeutic recreation services: On competence and outcomes.* State College, PA: Venture.

Stumbo, N. J., & Peterson, C. A. (2009). *Therapeutic recreation program design: Principles and procedures* (5th ed.). San Francisco: Benjamin Cummings.

Stumbo, N. J., & Wardlaw, B. (Eds.). (2011). *Facilitation of therapeutic recreation services: An evidence-based and best practice approach to techniques and processes.* State College, PA: Venture.

Sylvester, C., Voelkl, J. E., & Ellis, G. D. (2001). *Therapeutic recreation programming: Theory and practice.* State College, PA: Venture.

Tamparo, D. D., & Lewis, M. A. (2000). *Diseases of the human body* (3rd ed.). Philadelphia, PA: F. A. Davis Company.

Wilhite, B., & Keller, M. J. (2000). *Therapeutic recreation: Cases and exercises* (2nd ed.). State College, PA: Venture.

Recommended Books for Exam Preparation

American Therapeutic Recreation Association. (2009). *Code of ethics.* Alexandria, VA: Author.

American Therapeutic Recreation Association. (1998). *Finding the path: Ethics in action.* Hattiesburg, MS: Author. ISBN: 1-889435-13-9

American Therapeutic Recreation Association. (2000). *Standards for the practice of therapeutic recreation and self-assessment guide* (2nd ed.). Alexandria, VA: Author. ISBN: 1-889435-02-3

Austin, D. R. (2009). *Therapeutic recreation processes and techniques* (6th ed.). Urbana, IL: Sagamore. ISBN: 9781571675-47-7

Bullock, C. C., & Mahon, M. J. (2001). *Introduction to recreation services for people with disabilities: A person-centered approach.* Urbana, IL: Sagamore. ISBN: 1-57167-381-4

Burlingame, J., & Blaschko, T. M. (2010). *Assessment tools for recreational therapy* (3rd ed.). Ravensdale, WA: Idyll Arbor. ISBN: 9781882883721

Carter, M. J., & van Andel, G.E. (2010). *Therapeutic recreation: A practical approach* (4th ed.). Prospect Heights, IL: Waveland Press. ISBN:1577666-44-5

Carter, M. J., & O'Morrow, G. S. (2006). *Effective management in therapeutic recreation service.* (2nd ed.). State College, PA: Venture. ISBN: 1892132-62-1

Dattilo, J., & McKenney, A. (Eds.). (2011). *Facilitation techniques in therapeutic recreation* (2nd. ed.). State College, PA: Venture. ISBN: 1892132-93-1

Kunstler, R. & Daly, F. S. (2010). *Therapeutic recreation leadership and programming.* Champaign, IL: Human Kinetics. ISBN: 0736068-55-4

Mobily, K. E., & MacNeil, R. D. (2002). *Therapeutic recreation and the nature of disabilities.* State College, PA: Venture. ISBN: 1-892132-22-2

National Council for Therapeutic Recreation Certification. (2012). *Information for new applicants.* New City, NY: Author.

Stumbo, N. J. (2002). *Client assessment in therapeutic recreation services.* State College, PA: Venture. ISBN: 1-892132-32-x

Stumbo, N. J., & Peterson, C. A. (2009). *Therapeutic recreation program design: Principles and procedures* (5th ed.). San Francisco: Benjamin Cummings. ISBN:0805354-97-2

Stumbo, N. J., & Wardlaw, B. (Eds.). (2011). *Facilitation of therapeutic recreation services: An evidence-based and best practice approach to techniques and processes.* State College, PA: Venture. ISBN: 189213-29-4

chapter 5

Warm-Up Items

The 160 items that follow represent the types of questions included in the NCTRC national certification exam. The purpose of this warm-up is to give you some indication of the topics that will be covered, as well as to provide some additional questions for practice purposes. These questions do not represent the *proportion* of actual test questions within each of the Exam Content Outline categories. See Chapters 2 and 4 for more information about the proportion of items in each of the four categories on the actual test. For additional practice, six practice exams follow these warm-up items.

Directions: For each question in this section, select the BEST answer of the choices given. Use the answer scoring sheet on pages 76-77 to record your answers. Use the answer scoring key on page 78 to check your answers after you have completed all the items.

1. Which one of the four categories of child development does the skill "takes turns" belong?
    (A) Personal/social
    (B) Adaptive/fine motor behavior
    (C) Motor behavior
    (D) Language

2. Which of the following is NOT an example of a therapeutic recreation department's risk management plan?
    (A) Requiring TR student interns to complete their own client assessments
    (B) Requiring employees to park on hospital premises
    (C) Conducting peer reviews by trained professionals
    (D) Incorporating family into the assessment procedure

3. Which of the following activities is MOST LIKELY to teach social skills to a group of at-risk youth?
    (A) Bingo
    (B) Volleyball, because it involves both cooperation and competition
    (C) Role plays of asking someone for assistance
    (D) Discussion of appropriate leisure skills in a variety of situations

4. All of the following may be found in a therapeutic recreation department's policy and procedure manual, EXCEPT
    (A) instructions for checking out and driving agency vehicles
    (B) treatment protocols for disability groups served by the department
    (C) guidelines for prescribing medications
    (D) information about staff recruiting, hiring, supervision, and firing

5. The CTRS wants clients with severe intellectual disability to be able to freely choose their preferred leisure experiences. When the CTRS uses a variety of tactile, auditory, and gustatory objects from which the client chooses, it is called _____.
   (A) reality orientation
   (B) remotivation
   (C) assertiveness training
   (D) sensory stimulation

6. The CTRS uses the Transtheoretical Model of Behavior change in organizing her documentation on client behavior change. What are the "stages" of behavior change that she observes and documents on?
   (A) Thought, affect, behavior, evaluation
   (B) Rapid behavior change, slowed behavior change, and maintained behavior change
   (C) Precontemplation, contemplation, preparation, action, maintenance, and termination
   (D) Preparation, action, evaluation, and new action

7. Visualization can be helpful to clients because they can
   (A) use imaginary practice sessions for upcoming stressful situations
   (B) express their feelings without retribution from the group
   (C) relax at their own pace
   (D) only reveal to the group what they want to reveal

8. When using behavior modification with a female child who is emotionally disturbed, the CTRS teaches her separate hygiene behaviors (e.g., brushing her teeth, combing her hair) and then combines them altogether in a morning wake up routine. What behavior modification technique is the CTRS using?
   (A) Shaping
   (B) Modeling
   (C) Extinction
   (D) Chaining

9. The CTRS requires that all of her employees actively participate in diversity training on a regular basis. She is trying to ensure their _____ .
   (A) prejudices
   (B) cultural competence
   (C) attitudinal awareness
   (D) recertification through NCTRC

10. People with chronic pain may benefit from time management sessions because
    (A) they tend to be the busiest people
    (B) they tend to be complainers and procrastinators
    (C) it would help them identify goals for spending their least painful time constructively
    (D) it would help them develop a beneficial exercise routine at a local community center

11. Which of the following is NOT appropriate in the therapeutic recreation department's written plan of operation?
    (A) The mission, vision, and goals of the unit
    (B) Comprehensive and specific program protocols
    (C) The listing of assessments, evaluation, and their administrative procedures
    (D) Individual clients' treatment and program plans

12. A therapeutic recreation facilitation technique that focuses on taste, touch, sight, smell, hearing, and bodily movement, and is often combined with reminiscence and remotivation is called
    (A) sensory overload
    (B) aromatherapy
    (C) sensory stimulation
    (D) sensory integration

13. The CTRS is teaching clients with panic disorders to breathe from their diaphragms, rather than their chests, because
    (A) diaphragmatic breathing exchanges a greater volume of air
    (B) diaphragmatic breathing can leave the individual light headed
    (C) chest breathing is harder to learn
    (D) the activity analysis showed that more people would be successful

14. One of the primary components of a job description is the listing of
    (A) past work experiences
    (B) job duties to be performed
    (C) references
    (D) educational institutions attended

15. The CTRS is working with teenagers in a psychiatric inpatient program that is oriented toward Freudian psychology. One of the activities the CTRS would recommend for the clients based on "sublimation of sexual urges" is
(A) crafts
(B) a dance
(C) gymnastics
(D) tennis

16. Which one of the following activities is MOST LIKELY to aid a client in increased physical endurance?
(A) Leisure resource discussion group
(B) Video games
(C) Walking
(D) Yoga

17. Which of the following is the LEAST likely way for a CTRS to improve her continuing professional competence?
(A) Attend hospital grand rounds
(B) Present in-service training sessions to her colleagues
(C) Read brochures about services at similar facilities
(D) Attend national conferences

18. Which method of behavioral observation and recording is the CTRS using when she wants to record how often a behavior occurs during consecutive time periods?
(A) Frequency or tally
(B) Duration
(C) Interval
(D) Instantaneous time sampling

19. Which method of behavioral observation and recording is the CTRS using when she wants to record how long a client's outburst last??
(A) Frequency or tally
(B) Duration
(C) Interval
(D) Instantaneous time sampling

20. The best direct way to promote the value of therapeutic recreation services within a facility is to
(A) provide in-service trainings to other disciplines
(B) attend hospital grand rounds
(C) create and post an activity calendar on the unit
(D) create a multidisciplinary assessment

21. Which method of behavioral observation and recording is the CTRS using when he notes how many times the client uses negative self-statements?
(A) Frequency or tally
(B) Duration
(C) Interval
(D) Instantaneous time sampling

22. One method to increase inter-rater reliability in observations is to
(A) improve the construct validity of the instrument
(B) use clearly defined and non-overlapping categories
(C) support the results with extensive interviews
(D) purchase and compare similar interest inventories

23. All of the following are true statements about chronic pain EXCEPT
(A) chronic pain is defined as pain that lasts more than six months
(B) no major organic disorder can be found to explain chronic pain
(C) the typical onset of chronic pain is the age of 41
(D) chronic pain forms a cycle of lack of activity, then continued pain

24. Reality orientation is a technique used to combat what symptom(s)?
(A) Lack of assertiveness
(B) Irresponsibility and immaturity
(C) Chronic fatigue and stress
(D) Confusion

25. Using the following scenario, Client A is displaying which of the following types of behavior?

During a discussion on the value of leisure, Client A said, "We need to change topics. I don't like this one. I think it's for sissies like the rest of you guys." Client B said, "I feel like I'm benefiting from this discussion and I would like to continue." Client C said, "I'll go along with whatever the majority thinks."
(A) Assertive
(B) Nonassertive (passive)
(C) Aggressive
(D) Noncommittal

26. All of the following may be part of the department's risk management plan, EXCEPT
    (A) acceptable staff/client ratios for certain types of programs
    (B) qualifications and special certifications needed by staff
    (C) marketing brochures for fund raising purposes
    (D) procedures for reporting emergencies, crises, and critical incidents

27. The CTRS brought a wedding album, rice, a bridal veil, and a ring pillow to the session to trigger older adults to talk about their past experiences about weddings. What technique was the CTRS employing in this session?
    (A) Remotivation
    (B) Reality orientation
    (C) Reminiscence
    (D) Relaxation response

28. The modality of Remotivation includes all of the following EXCEPT
    (A) warm, caring, concerned environment
    (B) confrontation with other members of peer group
    (C) personal recollections of the topic of the day
    (D) connections between past and present reality

29. Which of the following medications is classified as an opioid?
    (A) Vicoden
    (B) Dexadrine
    (C) Tegretol
    (D) Naproxen

30. One of the principles in ATRA's Code of Ethics is Beneficience. This concept means
    (A) all individuals should receive identical services
    (B) all client have the basic right of self-determination
    (C) at best, provide benefit; at worst, do no harm
    (D) that confidentiality is expected in almost all situations

31. A CTRS is interested in determining a patient's leisure interests. From the following options, the CTRS should choose which assessment?
    (A) Leisure Diagnostic Battery (LDB)
    (B) Leisurescope
    (C) BANDI-RT
    (D) Comprehensive Evaluation in Recreational Therapy Scale (CERT) – Psych

32. The head of the therapeutic recreation department in a center that treats individuals who are addicted to opiods is likely to assure compliance with external accreditation standards?
    (A) Agency for Healthcare Research and Quality (AHRQ)
    (B) Rehabilitation Accreditation Commission (CARF)
    (C) Joint Commission (JCAHO)
    (D) Health Care Financing Administration (HCFA)

33. When appraising research for evidence-based practice, all of the following are appropriate questions EXCEPT
    (A) Do the results apply to my clients or situation?
    (B) Do the benefits outweigh any harm, costs, and/or inconveniences that are involved in the intervention?
    (C) What other factors need to be considered when applying this evidence?
    (D) Does the study report confidence intervals?

34. To be classified as legally blind, a person must have visual acuity no better than
    (A) 20/20
    (B) 10/200
    (C) 20/200
    (D) 10/100

35. Biofeedback, meditation, autogenic training, and progressive muscle relaxation are examples of what kind of therapeutic recreation facilitation technique?
    (A) Relaxation training
    (B) Tai chi
    (C) Guided imagery
    (D) Sensory stimulation

36. The CTRS is instructed to prepare a zero-based budget for the upcoming fiscal year. This means that the CTRS
    (A) adds a certain percentage to last year's budget to calculate this year's budget
    (B) receives no salary raise for the upcoming year
    (C) builds this year's budget from scratch
    (D) must negotiate with other departments to get more money in the budget

37. The primary reason the American Therapeutic Recreation Association was created in 1984 was to
    (A) provide services to veterans returning from the Vietnam War
    (B) provide workshops and conferences for members to get CEUs
    (C) create the national certification examination for therapeutic recreation specialists
    (D) respond to concerns and issues of therapeutic recreation specialists working in clinical facilities

38. The difference between an operational budget and a capital budget is that an operational budget
    (A) includes large expenditures of any kind over $500
    (B) covers all revenues and expenditures, except personnel
    (C) covers day-to-day revenues and expenditures for a one-year period
    (D) has line-items that can be vetoed by the agency president

39. Using the following scenario, Client B is displaying which of the following types of behavior?

    During a discussion on the value of leisure, Client A said, "We need to change topics. I don't like this one. I think it's for sissies like the rest of you guys." Client B said, " I feel like I'm benefiting from this discussion and I would like to continue." Client C said, "I'll go along with whatever the majority thinks."
    (A) Assertive
    (B) Nonassertive (passive)
    (C) Aggressive
    (D) Noncommittal

40. One of the major long-term effects of repeated use of inhalants is
    (A) extreme thirst
    (B) a strong reaction to sunlight
    (C) bruising of the forearms
    (D) improved sight acuity

41. Alcoholism is characterized by
    (A) physical dependence on alcohol and interruption in typical life functions
    (B) drinking 3-7 drinks per day
    (C) spending more than 20% of income on alcoholic beverages
    (D) repeated intoxication in public

42. Accreditation standards for ambulatory health care, behavioral health care, home care, and hospitals come from which of the following organizations?
    (A) Agency for Healthcare Research and Quality (AHRQ)
    (B) Commission on Accreditation of Rehabilitation Facilities (CARF)
    (C) Joint Commission (JCAHO)
    (D) Health Care Financing Administration (HCFA)

43. Feelings of overwhelming dread or impending doom with increased uneasiness are characteristics of
    (A) somatoform disorders
    (B) schizophrenia
    (C) anxiety disorders
    (D) multiple personality disorders

44. In order to teach adults appropriate social skills, the CTRS task analyzes the skill of "beginning a conversation with a new person." All of the additional techniques would be appropriate to teach social skills, EXCEPT
    (A) demonstration by the CTRS
    (B) practice and repetition by the client
    (C) practice with feedback from peers in the group
    (D) paper and pencil test

45. Managed care has shifted the responsibility of determining the services a patient needs from the providers of services to the_____.
    (A) state governments
    (B) payers of service
    (C) patient
    (D) middle class

46. In a prospective payment system of health care, the hospital knows that a specific amount will be paid by the insurance company for a particular surgery, regardless of the
    (A) skill of the surgeon
    (B) ethnicity of the patient
    (C) actual cost of the surgery
    (D) intended outcomes

47. Which of the following is MOST likely to produce positive attitudes toward individuals with disabilities?
(A) Increased exposure to and contact with individuals with disabilities
(B) Special discount rates to events and attractions
(C) Segregated or specialized services for individuals with disabilities
(D) Negative terminology and extensive classification systems

48. The organization that provides personnel standards for therapeutic recreation specialists is
(A) National Therapeutic Recreation Society (NTRS)
(B) American Therapeutic Recreation Association (ATRA)
(C) National Council for Therapeutic Recreation Certification (NCTRC)
(D) Joint Commission (JCAHO)

49. All of the following are examples of passive body language, EXCEPT
(A) erect body posture
(B) dropped head
(C) little eye contact
(D) hands kept in the lap

50. Which of the following federal acts defined therapeutic recreation as a related area of service and was responsible for allowing more people with disabilities to be served by CTRSs?
(A) 1973 Rehabilitation Act
(B) Smith-Sears Veterans Rehabilitation Act
(C) Individuals with Disabilities Education Act
(D) White House Conference on Handicapped Individuals Act

51. In the process of developing an assessment instrument, the CTRS observes and rates the client. Then the first CTRS has another CTRS observe and rate the client on the same functional behaviors. The ratings are then compared, with a nearly perfect coefficient. What instrument characteristic is being determined?
(A) Validity
(B) Reliability
(C) Usability
(D) Practicality

52. To receive the full benefits of a leisure experience, most CTRSs believe that the experience should be
(A) spontaneous
(B) motivational
(C) intrinsically motivated
(D) challenging

53. If a client assessment produces results that are reliable, it means that
(A) the content of the assessment matches the content of the intervention program
(B) the same client will receive about the same score if given the assessment twice
(C) clients are placed into the most appropriate programs to meet their needs
(D) two different assessments will produce the same results over time

54. A CTRS who works at a residential facility for at-risk youth, uses Piaget's Cognitive Theory of Development to develop age-appropriate activities. For the 2- to 7-year-olds, he specifically focuses on
(A) advanced language skills
(B) development of abstract reasoning
(C) symbolic play such as playing house or using puppets
(D) group consensus about the rules of games

55. Which of the following agencies is responsible for developing standards for facilities that serve individuals with spinal cord injuries, chronic pain, and traumatic brain injuries?
(A) American Therapeutic Recreation Association (ATRA)
(B) Joint Commission (JCAHO)
(C) Centers for Medicare and Medicaid Services (CMS)
(D) Rehabilitation Accreditation Commission (CARF)

56. All of the following would be principles of effective time management, EXCEPT
(A) minimize time wasters
(B) procrastinate at least once a day
(C) create an ongoing list of goals and priorities
(D) keep an organizer or calendar close at hand

57. If a facility does not meet standards and is not accredited by the Joint Commission (JCAHO) what is likely to be the result?
    (A) Medicare, Medicaid, and private insurance companies will not pay for services
    (B) The administration will seek accreditation by CARF
    (C) Staff's wages will be garnished until the problem is corrected
    (D) Nothing, accreditation by the Joint Commission (JCAHO) is not mandatory

58. One of the basic principles of assertiveness training is
    (A) if allowed, people will tend to be aggressive toward one another
    (B) that the majority of people need a significant amount of training in social skills
    (C) that each individual should be able to stand up for his/her rights, while acknowledging the rights of others
    (D) that most stress is experienced when trying to work with others

59. A CTRS who works with older adults in a long-term care facility, uses Erikson's Theory of Psychosocial Development to develop age- and stage-appropriate programs. Specifically she provides programs that help clients to
    (A) increase co-morbidities and secondary conditions
    (B) become more community-minded and less self-focused
    (C) meet their own needs through intrinsically motivated leisure
    (D) reconcile limits and losses associated with aging and mortality

60. All of the following assist individuals in coping with stress, EXCEPT their
    (A) attitudes of feeling challenged instead of threatened
    (B) feelings of having adequate resources to deal with the situation
    (C) Type A personalities
    (D) adequate social support networks

61. Which of the following best represents the theory of recreation substitutability?
    (A) The activity does not matter, it's the experience that counts
    (B) The second string squad often plays as well as the first string squad
    (C) Unable to do one activity, the person chooses another that provides similar satisfactions and benefits
    (D) There is no substitute for a person's favorite leisure activity so it must always be available

62. Stress management involves a variety of techniques, activities, and interventions designed to
    (A) reduce unfamiliar stress
    (B) cope more effectively with distress and add more positive stress (eustress)
    (C) increase the individual's capacity to take on and handle more stress
    (D) aid individuals who have recently suffered severe and significant losses

63. One of the most important ways in which CTRSs help clients develop independent and satisfying leisure lifestyles is by teaching them
    (A) as many leisure activities as possible
    (B) how to make positive leisure choices for self-involvement
    (C) how to access public transportation and leisure facilities
    (D) the concepts of self-determination and intrinsic motivation

64. The Comprehensive Evaluation in Recreation Therapy – Physical Disabilities (CERT-PD) measures which of the following sensory abilities EXCEPT
    (A) visual acuity
    (B) ocular pursuit
    (C) depth perception
    (D) taste perception

65. Which of the following is NOT assessed as part of a cognitive assessment for older adults?
    (A) Memory
    (B) Communication skills
    (C) Problem-solving skills
    (D) Safety awareness

66. Title II in the Americans with Disabilities Act of 1990 (and later amendments) concerns discrimination with regard to
(A) recreation services and facilities
(B) employment
(C) education
(D) both physical and programmatic access

67. Using the following scenario, Client C is displaying which of the following types of behavior?

During a discussion on the value of leisure, Client A said, "We need to change topics. I don't like this one. I think it's for sissies like the rest of you guys." Client B said, "I feel like I'm benefiting from this discussion and I would like to continue." Client C said, "I'll go along with whatever the majority thinks."
(A) Assertive
(B) Nonassertive (passive)
(C) Aggressive
(D) Noncommittal

68. Which of the following is listed as a related service under the Individuals with Disabilities Education Act of 2004?
(A) Therapeutic recreation
(B) Personal (exercise) training
(C) Science education
(D) Medicaid

69. The CTRS is leading a group of elderly clients who are disoriented using Validation Therapy. Which phase is being used when the CTRS says, "Sometimes I feel very lonely and when I do, I go looking for a friend. Do you ever feel lonely, Mrs. Jones?"
(A) Birth of the Group—Creating Energy
(B) Life of the Group—Verbal Interaction
(C) Movement and Rhythm
(D) Closing of the Group with Anticipation for the Next Meeting

70. Which of the following statements is NOT a suggested principle for structuring inclusionary programs?
(A) Exempt the person with the disability from rules that require physical or intellectual skill.
(B) Rotate positions and roles of the participants within the activity or program.
(C) Role model positive, accepting behavior as the leader of the activity or program.
(D) Accent positive attributes and skills of all participants.

71. What is the primary feature that distinguishes "therapeutic recreation" from "recreation?"
(A) Setting in which interventions takes place
(B) Purposeful nature of intervention to bring about behavioral change
(C) Nature of the selected experiences to facilitate outcomes
(D) Extent of time leaders prepare for interventions and follow-up after intervention

72. The term "continuity of care" means that the
(A) treatment team strives to provide predictable, connected, meaningful programs to clients
(B) client is transitioned from clinical to community settings
(C) client is involved in inclusive recreation services in the community with non-disabled peers
(D) specialist serves as a case manager throughout the client's length of stay at the facility

73. Which of the following statement are true about persons qualifying for services under the Individuals with Disabilities Education Act of 2004?
(A) All individuals aged 5 through 21 with disabilities qualify for services
(B) All individuals pre-school to age 21 with disabilities and with need qualify for services
(C) Only individuals with cognitive, emotional, and physical disabilities from pre-school to 21 qualify for services
(D) Only individuals with cognitive and physical disabilities who have an IQ above 85 qualify for services

74. Which question below addresses client evaluation?
(A) How consistent are the services being delivered to clients?
(B) How many programs did the client attend?
(C) Was the specialist effective and efficient in delivering intervention services to the client?
(D) What proposed outcomes were achieved as the result of the client's involvement in the program?

75. "Accessible" facilities become "usable" when the person with a disability can
(A) expect to receive special treatment and services
(B) function as independently as possible
(C) socialize with individuals with similar disabilities
(D) enter through the front door and use the restroom area

76. The CTRS tracks the number of times a client responds appropriately to another peer, in order to monitor the effects of the social skills program. This type of observation is being recorded through the _____ method.
    (A) tally
    (B) duration
    (C) interval
    (D) instantaneous time sampling

77. Utilization review in hospitals is the process of
    (A) recruiting, interviewing and hiring new specialists from various disciplines
    (B) changing from retrospective payments to managed care
    (C) evaluating the most efficient and effective use of resources
    (D) making sure all professionals attend professional conferences in their discipline

78. The purpose of an assessment protocol is to
    (A) make sure every client has the same diagnosis and treatment plan
    (B) increase sensitivity to cultural minorities
    (C) align the therapeutic recreation assessment with the occupational therapy assessment
    (D) increase the reliability of the assessment administration

79. What piece of legislation mandates program accessibility in public accommodations?
    (A) Americans with Disabilities Act of 1990
    (B) Section 504 of the 1973 Vocational Rehabilitation Amendments
    (C) Architectural Barriers Act of 1968
    (D) Public Law 94-142 of 1975

80. The CTRS wants the client to gain upper body strength so he can propel his wheelchair for longer distances. The CTRS would MOST LIKELY use
    (A) weight training
    (B) wheelchair basketball
    (C) Tai Chi
    (D) anaerobic exercise

81. According to *Healthy People 2020*, individuals with disabilities are more likely to experience poorer health than their non-disabled counterparts because all of the following EXCEPT
    (A) inaccessibility of health care facilities
    (B) inaccessibility of physical fitness areas and facilities
    (C) lack of social support
    (D) improved health care monitoring

82. The Functional Assessment of Characteristics for Therapeutic Recreation – Revised (FACTR-R) measures which of the following?
    (A) Leisure functioning
    (B) Decision-making skills
    (C) Prerequisite skills related to leisure participation
    (D) Leisure skills typically needed to live in the community

83. A "leisure lifestyle" means that the individual
    (A) is unemployed and is "at leisure" for most of the day
    (B) has developed a daily pattern of leisure involvement
    (C) participates in a variety of leisure activities
    (D) is independent in most if not all of daily activities

84. Which of the following is NOT assessed as part of a social skills assessment for youth in psychiatric treatment?
    (A) Tell me how you would introduce yourself to a youth you didn't know.
    (B) Where is a good place to meet other kids with common leisure interests?
    (C) How would you ask someone to go bowling with you?
    (D) When was the last time you played a game for more than 30 minutes?

85. All of the following are examples of physical benefits of leisure participation EXCEPT
    (A) potential counteragent to negative lifestyle choices
    (B) reduction of secondary disabilities
    (C) improved health indicators such as bone density and joint mobility
    (D) increase in high blood pressure and heart disease

86. Which of the following activities is most likely based on competition?
    (A) Scrabble
    (B) Dancing
    (C) Dramatic theatre
    (D) Running

87. Which of the following is an example of a "structure" indicator in therapeutic recreation services?
    (A) Proportion of therapeutic recreation specialists to other therapists
    (B) Outcomes of clients who receive therapeutic recreation services
    (C) Frequency of interactions between clients and therapists
    (D) Client achievement of social interaction skills objectives

88. As the level of intellectual disability increases from mild to severe/profound, the CTRS should expect to see increased
    (A) social and intellectual skill development
    (B) compensation for skill deficits
    (C) need for transportation
    (D) secondary physical limitations and sensory impairments

89. Time management is the practice of
    (A) structuring time to focus on important activities and minimizing unimportant activities
    (B) fitting more activities into a person's schedule
    (C) reducing the number of com'itments on your time
    (D) keeping track of events and appointments in a personal calendar

90. Typical treatment for a decubitus ulcer includes
    (A) increased cardiovascular exercise
    (B) a prescription for blood pressure medicine
    (C) bed rest and antibiotics
    (D) daily stress management classes

91. Which of the following is an example of as "outcome" indicator in therapeutic recreation services?
    (A) Proportion of therapeutic recreation specialists to other therapists
    (B) Proportion of clients who receive therapeutic recreation services
    (C) Proportion of clients treated according to therapeutic recreation protocols
    (D) Client achievement of social interaction skills objectives

92. The client is showing signs of disorientation, confusion and memory loss. After the CTRS completes the assessment and meets with the treatment team, he/she should use which of the following intervention techniques?
    (A) Resocialization
    (B) Remotivation
    (C) Reality orientation
    (D) Refocusing

93. The CTRS provides many active games and sports to adolescents with emotional disturbances to allow for the release of disorganized and pent-up emotions. The CTRS adheres to which of the following theories of play?
    (A) Custodial
    (B) Psychoanalytical
    (C) Compensatory
    (D) Catharsis

94. The CTRS designed a program to assist older adults with intellectual disability to share their previous life experiences after reading poetry about children. The CTRS was using a technique known as _____.
    (A) reality orientation
    (B) remotivation
    (C) teach back
    (D) cognitive restructuring

95. A client's sense of control may be increased through all the following ways EXCEPT
    (A) asking what type of community event the person would like to attend
    (B) giving the client an important role in planning to attend the event
    (C) asking the client to take part in the meal preparation
    (D) placing the sign-up sheet in the main activity room so all can find it

96. The CTRS, in an assertiveness training session, teaches clients to avoid being persuaded by others into doing something against their wishes, by repeating a concise statement of refusal. The CTRS is teaching clients the technique of
    (A) clouding
    (B) broken record
    (C) compromise
    (D) defusing

97. An advantage of calling someone's references before hiring him is that the supervisor can
    (A) ask the reference to compare qualifications of several applicants
    (B) ask about personal issues such as family status, drug and alcohol history, and religion
    (C) verify information from the resume or interview
    (D) orient the employee to hospital procedures and introduce staff of different departments

98. In order to benefit from aerobic exercise, individuals need to reach and stay within their target heart rate for at least twenty minutes. This formula for calculating target heart rate is
    (A) age minus 20, times 1.5
    (B) 60 to 75 percent of normal maximum heart rate
    (C) weight minus 15, plus age
    (D) 40 percent of normal maximum heart rate

99. The Centers for Medicare and Medicaid Services (CMS) monitors quality assessment and performance improvement in facilities that
    (A) serve individuals covered by the federal government's health insurance program
    (B) use the Therapeutic Recreation Accountability Model
    (C) adhere to the American Therapeutic Recreation Association's Standards of Practice
    (D) are located in low-income, urban areas

100. In the following exchange, Client A was showing which of the following behavioral styles?

    A: "You guys must cover for me when the head nurse comes and asks why I wasn't in group therapy this morning." B: "Okay, whatever you say." C: "No, I can't do that for you, because that would be lying."
    (A) Aggressive
    (B) Passive
    (C) Assertive
    (D) Emotive

101. Which of the following is an example of a program based on the principle of "normalization?"
    (A) Older adults with sensory deficits are taken to a playground.
    (B) Female teenagers with intellectual disabilities play video games and listen to music.
    (C) Youths in juvenile detention attend programs on vacationing overseas.
    (D) All children with disabilities are registered for community recreation programs.

102. The CTRS employs an activity that focuses on the client's thoughts. What is this kind of therapy called?
    (A) Cognitive therapy
    (B) Behavior therapy
    (C) Affective therapy
    (D) Gestalt therapy

103. Which of the following is an example of intrinsically motivated leisure?
    (A) The client joins a quilters club for her own enjoyment
    (B) The client's incentive for joining the running club is the trophies
    (C) The client learns golf so he can play golf with his colleagues
    (D) The client joined the fitness center because many of his friends are members

104. The CTRS has clients discuss whether their daily behavior reflects their statements that their own personal health is of high importance. The specialist is using which of the following therapeutic recreation facilitation techniques?
    (A) Bibliotherapy
    (B) Remotivation
    (C) Resocialization
    (D) Values clarification

105. The CTRS is aware that clients, like the rest of the American population, are apt to be more overweight and obese, and he realizes this puts them at risk of not having a healthy and satisfying leisure lifestyle. To find out information about this trend as well as ways to reverse it, the CTRS should read documents at which of the following web sites?
    (A) www.toofatforhealth.org
    (B) www.healthypeople.gov
    (C) www.takebackyourtime.org
    (D) www.recreationtherapy.com

106. The CTRS is leading a group of elderly clients who are disoriented using Validation Therapy. Which phase is being used when the CTRS says, "Mr. Smith did you remember to bring the poem you wanted to share with us? You did. Great! O.K., let's listen to Mr. Smith's poem."
    (A) Birth of the Group—Creating Energy
    (B) Life of the Group—Verbal Interaction
    (C) Movement and Rhythm
    (D) Closing of the Group with Anticipation for the Next Meeting

107. In developing a leisure lifestyle, an individual often selects leisure experiences in which they can expect reasonable success, based on past experiences and past success. This is based on the concept of
    (A) self-determination
    (B) ecological development
    (C) perceived competence
    (D) optimal functioning

108. When a CTRS provides an accepting and understanding attitude to a client and, as a result, that positive involvement reduces the client's feelings of loneliness and worthlessness, and helps the client to take responsibility to alter irresponsible behavior, the CTRS is probably using what therapy?
    (A) Psychoanalytic
    (B) Behavior
    (C) Reality
    (D) Rational emotive

109. Medicare Part A provides for all of the following health services EXCEPT
    (A) in-patient hospital care
    (B) skilled nursing in long-term care
    (C) hospice care
    (D) outpatient rehabilitation services

110. Which of the following activity titles seem MOST appropriate to help clients develop social skills?
    (A) Bingo
    (B) Interaction skills for adults
    (C) Low-cost activities for children
    (D) Volleyball

111. The CTRS is leading a group of elderly clients who are disoriented using Validation Therapy. In which phase does the CTRS serve refreshments and plays an upbeat song?
    (A) Birth of the Group—Creating Energy
    (B) Life of the Group—Verbal Interaction
    (C) Movement and Rhythm
    (D) Closing of the Group with Anticipation for the Next Meeting

112. The CTRS met one of her client's relatives in a local restaurant and let them know that his prescriptions had recently been changed to better control his behavior. The CTRS violated provisions in the
    (A) Medicaid and Medicare regulations
    (B) Older Americans Act of 1965 and its reauthorizations
    (C) Health Insurance Portability and Accountability Act (HIPAA) of 1996
    (D) Patient Privacy Act (PPA) of 2010

113. Considering the typical leisure patterns of adolescents, which activity choice is MOST LIKELY to be appropriate?
    (A) Community folk and social dance club
    (B) Square dancing
    (C) Computer and video games
    (D) Crossword puzzles

114. The Analysis part of a SOAP note contains what types of information?
    (A) Assessment
    (B) Activity recommendations
    (C) Interpretation of data
    (D) Revisions in the treatment plan

115. In Rational Emotive Therapy, the focus is placed on
    (A) irrational self-statements that interfere with a person's ability to see reality objectively
    (B) reducing stress by eliminating emotions that are not rational
    (C) paying attention to the physiological responses to stress
    (D) clarifying what the person thinks or feels about his or her family members

116. An advantage of SOAP notes over narrative notes is that they
    (A) are completed only by select members of the treatment team
    (B) contain more subjective information about the client
    (C) are more structured and organized
    (D) require behavioral observations

117. When he is upset or things do not go his way, the client lashes out at people, often making very caustic remarks and sometimes striking them. A therapeutic recreation facilitation technique that is MOST LIKELY to help the client is called
    (A) journaling
    (B) reality therapy
    (C) resocialization
    (D) anger management

118. Which of the following is a formative program evaluation question?
    (A) What unanticipated events or outcomes occurred in this program that were not part of the program plan?
    (B) Did the sequence of activities appear to be logical and appropriate?
    (C) How much time will be allotted for the program next time it is offered?
    (D) Are there enough resources for the remainder of the program?

119. If a person believes that he/she does not have the right skills to complete a leisure experience, and then generalized this inadequacy to all other leisure behaviors, this person is exhibiting which of the following?
    (A) Leisure efficacy
    (B) Learned helplessness
    (C) Attributional leisure response
    (D) Extrinsic motivation

120. When is it most appropriate to use structured observations for client assessment?
    (A) When actual behavior is of concern
    (B) When the person's perceptions of behaviors are important
    (C) When the person acts out in public
    (D) Rarely, interviews are always the better choice for client assessment purposes

121. Which of the following is NOT appropriate to document in the therapeutic recreation department's written plan of operation?
    (A) The philosophy of the therapeutic recreation department
    (B) Comprehensive and specific program descriptions
    (C) Description of assessment tool and assessment protocol
    (D) The treatment plans and progress notes

122. Meditation is the practice of
    (A) resolving domestic violence conflicts
    (B) attempting to mindfully focus on one thought at a time
    (C) chanting mantras while in a yoga position
    (D) making clients responsible for their own behaviors

123. Knowing the payer mix of the agency is important because it
    (A) influences how external accreditation agencies review the various departments
    (B) requires an extensive knowledge of insurance company forms
    (C) influences how the agency gets reimbursed for services
    (D) shortens the patient's length of stay

124. Which of the following is an example of a probe that could be used during a client assessment?
    (A) "My name is Reginald and I'd like to learn as much as I can today about your leisure"
    (B) "To summarize your comments thus far...."
    (C) "And now let's move to the third section of the assessment..."
    (D) "Tell me more about your artistic ability"

125. The process by which a nongovernmental agency or association grants recognition to an individual who has met certain predetermined qualifications specified by that agency or association is called
    (A) licensure
    (B) accreditation
    (C) certification
    (D) registration

126. Biofeedback can help individuals learn to modify all of the following bodily functions, EXCEPT
    (A) muscle tension
    (B) skin surface temperature
    (C) blood pressure
    (D) rapid eye movement

127. The process by which qualified individuals are listed on an official roster maintained by a governmental or non-governmental agency is called
    (A) licensure
    (B) accreditation
    (C) certification
    (D) registration

128. Which of the following represents the highest level of cross-cultural competence?
    (A) Being aware that one is lacking knowledge about another culture
    (B) Learning about clients' cultures and providing culturally specific interventions
    (C) Automatically providing culturally congruent care to clients of diverse cultures
    (D) Not being aware that one is lacking knowledge about another culture

129. The CTRS wants to assess whether her clients follow the American College of Sports Medicine guidelines for physical activity involvement. She asks which of the following questions?
    (A) Do you, on average, exercise for 30 minutes per day at least 5 days a week?
    (B) Do you participate in at least 4 physical leisure activities per week?
    (C) Do you achieve a resting heart rate of at least 100 beats per minute?
    (D) How many miles do you walk in one day, on average?

130. Managed care is an effort on behalf of insurance companies to
    (A) increase patient's length of stay
    (B) control costs of caring for clients
    (C) reduce the paperwork involved in client care
    (D) decrease the number of preferred provider organizations (PPOs)

131. The Health Insurance Portability and Accountability Act (HIPAA) of 1996 and its updates provide which of the following for health care recipients?
    (A) States must have 'reciprocity' for employee health insurance plans
    (B) Information about an individual's health care is protected from unwarranted disclosure
    (C) All recipients must have access to the results of quality improvement efforts of their health care providers
    (D) Health insurance policies must be transferable between employment settings

132. Which of the following types of activity often is used in stress management programs?
    (A) Progressive muscle relaxation
    (B) Remotivation
    (C) Social skills training
    (D) Trust building

133. For a service to be reimbursable, in many instances insurance companies require the therapist to provide what information or evidence?
    (A) Assessment tools sanctioned by JCAHO, HCFA, or CARF
    (B) Source-oriented medical records
    (C) Physician's orders
    (D) Risk management plan for the activity

134. An "optimal experience" (commonly called a peak experience or flow) is more likely to happen when
    (A) the person's skills are adequate for the challenge
    (B) the individual is surrounded by loved ones
    (C) it is preceded by pleasant emotions and positive regard
    (D) the person is highly skilled at the activity

135. Which of the following assessments would be located in the category of Leisure Attitudes and Barriers?
    (A) Leisure Motivation Scale (LMS)
    (B) BANDI-RT
    (C) Therapeutic Recreation Index (TRI)
    (D) Global Assessment of Functioning (GAF)

136. Evaluation is conducted on specific individual programs in order to
    (A) provide systematic information for future program decisions
    (B) provide systematic information on client regression
    (C) increase validity and reliability of client assessment procedures
    (D) develop individual client treatment plans

137. Which of the following is an important premise of Reality Therapy?
    (A) The specialist helps the client stay oriented to time, person and place
    (B) The client is responsible for all of his or her behavior
    (C) The specialist helps the client explore connections between past experiences and present actions
    (D) The specialist helps the client focus on stopping irrational thoughts

138. Which of the following is NOT a condition of informed consent?
    (A) Person is capable of making health care decisions
    (B) Person is acting voluntarily without coercion or deceit
    (C) Person has immediate access to health care records
    (D) Person is provided simple yet complete information about the procedures, risks, benefits, and alternatives

139. The client says that involvement with her family is very important to her, but spends an inordinate amount of time at work, usually bringing home a large pile of work to do in the evenings and on the weekends. The CTRS may use what type of therapeutic technique to help her review her priorities and behaviors?
    (A) Values clarification
    (B) Reality orientation
    (C) Assertiveness training
    (D) Bibliotherapy

140. Cataracts involve clouding of the cornea of the eyeball and is the leading cause of
    (A) falls in the elderly
    (B) blindness
    (C) glaucoma
    (D) nearsightedness

141. Which of the following is an appropriate program evaluation question to ask clients?
    (A) How satisfied were you with the qualifications of the staff?
    (B) What did you learn from your participation in this program?
    (C) How do you spend your time with family?
    (D) How satisfied were you with the activity analysis of this program?

142. Which of the following is the BEST example of a receptive communication dysfunction?
    (A) Inability to transform experiences into language
    (B) Inability to comprehend the written or spoken word
    (C) Inability to express oneself through actions or language
    (D) Inability to distinguish nuances in spoken language

143. The process by which an agency or organization evaluates and recognizes a program of study or an institution as meeting certain predetermined qualifications or standards is called _____.
    (A) licensure
    (B) accreditation
    (C) certification
    (D) registration

144. Which of the following might be an outcome indicator assessed through a continuous quality improvement program?
    (A) Qualifications of the TR staff
    (B) Environment in which treatment is provided
    (C) Intervention strategies employed by the CTRS
    (D) Changes in the client's functional capacity

145. In the following exchange, Client B was showing which of the following behavioral styles?
    A: "I want you both to cover for me when the head nurse comes and asks why I wasn't in group therapy this morning."
    B: "Okay, whatever you say."
    C: "No, I can't do that for you, because that would be lying."
    (A) Aggressive
    (B) Passive
    (C) Assertive
    (D) Emotive

146. "Clinical indicators" are used in quality improvement to
    (A) evaluate the degree of client satisfaction with services received
    (B) compare one discipline's outcomes compared to other disciplines
    (C) measure how well the targets were achieved
    (D) provide a basis for evidence-based practice

147. In the following exchange, Client C was showing which of the following behavioral styles?
    A: "I want you both to cover for me when the head nurse comes and asks why I wasn't in group therapy this morning."
    B: "Okay, whatever you say."
    C: "No, I can't do that for you, because that would be lying."
    (A) Aggressive
    (B) Passive
    (C) Assertive
    (D) Emotive

148. The process of comparing the quantity of services provided with the amount of resources such as staff and time used is called
    (A) market segmenting
    (B) risk management
    (C) productivity measurement
    (D) analysis of care

149. Why does "thought stopping" help reduce stress reactions in people who have obsessive or phobic thoughts?
    (A) Thoughts precede emotions which precede physiological responses.
    (B) It punishes them for their negative thoughts.
    (C) It isolates them from the group before they can be hurt.
    (D) It shows them they have value and worth.

150. One of the primary tenets of the Health Insurance Portability and Accountability Act (HIPAA) of 1996 and later rules is that individual health information:
    (A) must be kept private and confidential
    (B) must be kept electronically so it can be shared with other providers
    (C) should be part of the individual's medical record
    (D) should be checked annually for medical errors

151. Which of the following is the BEST example of using guided visualization as a facilitation technique in therapeutic recreation?
    (A) Having a person with cancer imagine good cells chomping on cancerous cells
    (B) Asking a group to role play what they might do when a stranger approaches
    (C) Asking a group of clients to express their feelings through any visual art medium
    (D) Asking a client to paint a picture of her future leisure

152. Which statement describes an intent or purpose common to both systems planning and quality improvement plans?
    (A) Each describes the relationship of the comprehensive program to individual treatment plans
    (B) Each outlines the relationship between the agency and departmental procedures
    (C) Both define the components of department programs
    (D) Each provides a systematic method to evaluate service delivery

153. One example of a "trigger" within the Activities section on the MDS 3.0 would be when the individual
    (A) prefers more or different activity choices than are now being offered
    (B) rarely receives visits from family or friends
    (C) is completely independent in his/her leisure pursuits
    (D) is ready for discharge to his/her home

154. One document within a written plan of operation is the department's or unit's scope of care. The scope of care specifies
    (A) the comprehensive goals and program areas of the department
    (B) methods of treating groups of clients
    (C) the treatment protocols for specific diagnostic groups
    (D) how the CTRS should interact with the clients

155. In assessment the most significant source of information is usually the
    (A) client
    (B) care giver
    (C) medical records
    (D) team members

156. The following is an example of which one of the following health care delivery systems?
The focus of care is on the improvement of knowledge for the world of work.
    (A) Medical
    (B) Custodial
    (C) Milieu
    (D) Education and Training

157. A CTRS is nonjudgmental, nondirective, and provides an accepting atmosphere allowing the client to assume the same positive self-regard the CTRS has shown to the client. The CTRS is using _____ therapy.
    (A) gestalt
    (B) reality
    (C) rational emotive
    (D) person centered

158. From assessment results, the CTRS determines that the client has an inability to assert himself with peers or to follow through with commitments. He also lacks receptive communication skills. Which of the following therapeutic recreation programs would be MOST appropriate for this client?
    (A) Leisure planning
    (B) Social skills training
    (C) Leisure values and attitudes
    (D) Leisure resources

159. All of the following areas of a TR department's written plan of operation may have specific, written policies and procedures, EXCEPT
    (A) obtaining physician's orders for treatment of clients
    (B) employee hiring and firing procedures
    (C) how CTRSs apply for recertification
    (D) procedures for obtaining supplies from the dietary department

160. Which of the following is of primary importance for the CTRS to consider when selecting an intervention program that will produce a specific client outcome?
    (A) Resources necessary to offer the experiences
    (B) Staff skills needed to lead the activity
    (C) Functional requirements of the activity
    (D) Risk management protocols for the experience

Warm-up Items Scoring Sheet

1. Ⓐ Ⓑ Ⓒ Ⓓ	22. Ⓐ Ⓑ Ⓒ Ⓓ	43. Ⓐ Ⓑ Ⓒ Ⓓ	64. Ⓐ Ⓑ Ⓒ Ⓓ
2. Ⓐ Ⓑ Ⓒ Ⓓ	23. Ⓐ Ⓑ Ⓒ Ⓓ	44. Ⓐ Ⓑ Ⓒ Ⓓ	65. Ⓐ Ⓑ Ⓒ Ⓓ
3. Ⓐ Ⓑ Ⓒ Ⓓ	24. Ⓐ Ⓑ Ⓒ Ⓓ	45. Ⓐ Ⓑ Ⓒ Ⓓ	66. Ⓐ Ⓑ Ⓒ Ⓓ
4. Ⓐ Ⓑ Ⓒ Ⓓ	25. Ⓐ Ⓑ Ⓒ Ⓓ	46. Ⓐ Ⓑ Ⓒ Ⓓ	67. Ⓐ Ⓑ Ⓒ Ⓓ
5. Ⓐ Ⓑ Ⓒ Ⓓ	26. Ⓐ Ⓑ Ⓒ Ⓓ	47. Ⓐ Ⓑ Ⓒ Ⓓ	68. Ⓐ Ⓑ Ⓒ Ⓓ
6. Ⓐ Ⓑ Ⓒ Ⓓ	27. Ⓐ Ⓑ Ⓒ Ⓓ	48. Ⓐ Ⓑ Ⓒ Ⓓ	69. Ⓐ Ⓑ Ⓒ Ⓓ
7. Ⓐ Ⓑ Ⓒ Ⓓ	28. Ⓐ Ⓑ Ⓒ Ⓓ	49. Ⓐ Ⓑ Ⓒ Ⓓ	70. Ⓐ Ⓑ Ⓒ Ⓓ
8. Ⓐ Ⓑ Ⓒ Ⓓ	29. Ⓐ Ⓑ Ⓒ Ⓓ	50. Ⓐ Ⓑ Ⓒ Ⓓ	71. Ⓐ Ⓑ Ⓒ Ⓓ
9. Ⓐ Ⓑ Ⓒ Ⓓ	30. Ⓐ Ⓑ Ⓒ Ⓓ	51. Ⓐ Ⓑ Ⓒ Ⓓ	72. Ⓐ Ⓑ Ⓒ Ⓓ
10. Ⓐ Ⓑ Ⓒ Ⓓ	31. Ⓐ Ⓑ Ⓒ Ⓓ	52. Ⓐ Ⓑ Ⓒ Ⓓ	73. Ⓐ Ⓑ Ⓒ Ⓓ
11. Ⓐ Ⓑ Ⓒ Ⓓ	32. Ⓐ Ⓑ Ⓒ Ⓓ	53. Ⓐ Ⓑ Ⓒ Ⓓ	74. Ⓐ Ⓑ Ⓒ Ⓓ
12. Ⓐ Ⓑ Ⓒ Ⓓ	33. Ⓐ Ⓑ Ⓒ Ⓓ	54. Ⓐ Ⓑ Ⓒ Ⓓ	75. Ⓐ Ⓑ Ⓒ Ⓓ
13. Ⓐ Ⓑ Ⓒ Ⓓ	34. Ⓐ Ⓑ Ⓒ Ⓓ	55. Ⓐ Ⓑ Ⓒ Ⓓ	76. Ⓐ Ⓑ Ⓒ Ⓓ
14. Ⓐ Ⓑ Ⓒ Ⓓ	35. Ⓐ Ⓑ Ⓒ Ⓓ	56. Ⓐ Ⓑ Ⓒ Ⓓ	77. Ⓐ Ⓑ Ⓒ Ⓓ
15. Ⓐ Ⓑ Ⓒ Ⓓ	36. Ⓐ Ⓑ Ⓒ Ⓓ	57. Ⓐ Ⓑ Ⓒ Ⓓ	78. Ⓐ Ⓑ Ⓒ Ⓓ
16. Ⓐ Ⓑ Ⓒ Ⓓ	37. Ⓐ Ⓑ Ⓒ Ⓓ	58. Ⓐ Ⓑ Ⓒ Ⓓ	79. Ⓐ Ⓑ Ⓒ Ⓓ
17. Ⓐ Ⓑ Ⓒ Ⓓ	38. Ⓐ Ⓑ Ⓒ Ⓓ	59. Ⓐ Ⓑ Ⓒ Ⓓ	80. Ⓐ Ⓑ Ⓒ Ⓓ
18. Ⓐ Ⓑ Ⓒ Ⓓ	39. Ⓐ Ⓑ Ⓒ Ⓓ	60. Ⓐ Ⓑ Ⓒ Ⓓ	81. Ⓐ Ⓑ Ⓒ Ⓓ
19. Ⓐ Ⓑ Ⓒ Ⓓ	40. Ⓐ Ⓑ Ⓒ Ⓓ	61. Ⓐ Ⓑ Ⓒ Ⓓ	82. Ⓐ Ⓑ Ⓒ Ⓓ
20. Ⓐ Ⓑ Ⓒ Ⓓ	41. Ⓐ Ⓑ Ⓒ Ⓓ	62. Ⓐ Ⓑ Ⓒ Ⓓ	83. Ⓐ Ⓑ Ⓒ Ⓓ
21. Ⓐ Ⓑ Ⓒ Ⓓ	42. Ⓐ Ⓑ Ⓒ Ⓓ	63. Ⓐ Ⓑ Ⓒ Ⓓ	84. Ⓐ Ⓑ Ⓒ Ⓓ

85. Ⓐ Ⓑ Ⓒ Ⓓ
86. Ⓐ Ⓑ Ⓒ Ⓓ
87. Ⓐ Ⓑ Ⓒ Ⓓ
88. Ⓐ Ⓑ Ⓒ Ⓓ
89. Ⓐ Ⓑ Ⓒ Ⓓ
90. Ⓐ Ⓑ Ⓒ Ⓓ
91. Ⓐ Ⓑ Ⓒ Ⓓ
92. Ⓐ Ⓑ Ⓒ Ⓓ
93. Ⓐ Ⓑ Ⓒ Ⓓ
94. Ⓐ Ⓑ Ⓒ Ⓓ
95. Ⓐ Ⓑ Ⓒ Ⓓ
96. Ⓐ Ⓑ Ⓒ Ⓓ
97. Ⓐ Ⓑ Ⓒ Ⓓ
98. Ⓐ Ⓑ Ⓒ Ⓓ
99. Ⓐ Ⓑ Ⓒ Ⓓ
100. Ⓐ Ⓑ Ⓒ Ⓓ
101. Ⓐ Ⓑ Ⓒ Ⓓ
102. Ⓐ Ⓑ Ⓒ Ⓓ
103. Ⓐ Ⓑ Ⓒ Ⓓ

104. Ⓐ Ⓑ Ⓒ Ⓓ
105. Ⓐ Ⓑ Ⓒ Ⓓ
106. Ⓐ Ⓑ Ⓒ Ⓓ
107. Ⓐ Ⓑ Ⓒ Ⓓ
108. Ⓐ Ⓑ Ⓒ Ⓓ
109. Ⓐ Ⓑ Ⓒ Ⓓ
110. Ⓐ Ⓑ Ⓒ Ⓓ
111. Ⓐ Ⓑ Ⓒ Ⓓ
112. Ⓐ Ⓑ Ⓒ Ⓓ
113. Ⓐ Ⓑ Ⓒ Ⓓ
114. Ⓐ Ⓑ Ⓒ Ⓓ
115. Ⓐ Ⓑ Ⓒ Ⓓ
116. Ⓐ Ⓑ Ⓒ Ⓓ
117. Ⓐ Ⓑ Ⓒ Ⓓ
118. Ⓐ Ⓑ Ⓒ Ⓓ
119. Ⓐ Ⓑ Ⓒ Ⓓ
120. Ⓐ Ⓑ Ⓒ Ⓓ
121. Ⓐ Ⓑ Ⓒ Ⓓ
122. Ⓐ Ⓑ Ⓒ Ⓓ

123. Ⓐ Ⓑ Ⓒ Ⓓ
124. Ⓐ Ⓑ Ⓒ Ⓓ
125. Ⓐ Ⓑ Ⓒ Ⓓ
126. Ⓐ Ⓑ Ⓒ Ⓓ
127. Ⓐ Ⓑ Ⓒ Ⓓ
128. Ⓐ Ⓑ Ⓒ Ⓓ
129. Ⓐ Ⓑ Ⓒ Ⓓ
130. Ⓐ Ⓑ Ⓒ Ⓓ
131. Ⓐ Ⓑ Ⓒ Ⓓ
132. Ⓐ Ⓑ Ⓒ Ⓓ
133. Ⓐ Ⓑ Ⓒ Ⓓ
134. Ⓐ Ⓑ Ⓒ Ⓓ
135. Ⓐ Ⓑ Ⓒ Ⓓ
136. Ⓐ Ⓑ Ⓒ Ⓓ
137. Ⓐ Ⓑ Ⓒ Ⓓ
138. Ⓐ Ⓑ Ⓒ Ⓓ
139. Ⓐ Ⓑ Ⓒ Ⓓ
140. Ⓐ Ⓑ Ⓒ Ⓓ
141. Ⓐ Ⓑ Ⓒ Ⓓ

142. Ⓐ Ⓑ Ⓒ Ⓓ
143. Ⓐ Ⓑ Ⓒ Ⓓ
144. Ⓐ Ⓑ Ⓒ Ⓓ
145. Ⓐ Ⓑ Ⓒ Ⓓ
146. Ⓐ Ⓑ Ⓒ Ⓓ
147. Ⓐ Ⓑ Ⓒ Ⓓ
148. Ⓐ Ⓑ Ⓒ Ⓓ
149. Ⓐ Ⓑ Ⓒ Ⓓ
150. Ⓐ Ⓑ Ⓒ Ⓓ
151. Ⓐ Ⓑ Ⓒ Ⓓ
152. Ⓐ Ⓑ Ⓒ Ⓓ
153. Ⓐ Ⓑ Ⓒ Ⓓ
154. Ⓐ Ⓑ Ⓒ Ⓓ
155. Ⓐ Ⓑ Ⓒ Ⓓ
156. Ⓐ Ⓑ Ⓒ Ⓓ
157. Ⓐ Ⓑ Ⓒ Ⓓ
158. Ⓐ Ⓑ Ⓒ Ⓓ
159. Ⓐ Ⓑ Ⓒ Ⓓ
160. Ⓐ Ⓑ Ⓒ Ⓓ

Warm-Up Items Scoring Key

Foundational Knowledge

1. A	40. A	59. D	75. B	93. D	112. C
6. C	41. A	61. C	79. A	95. D	119. B
9. B	43. C	63. B	81. D	101. B	128. C
15. B	47. A	66. D	83. B	103. A	131. B
23. C	50. C	68. A	85. D	105. B	134. A
29. A	52. C	70. A	88. D	107. C	140. B
34. C	54. C	73. B	90. C	109. D	142. B
					156. D

Practice of TR/RT

3. C	24. D	56. B	80. A	106. A	132. A
5. D	25. C	58. C	82. C	108. D	135. A
7. A	27. C	60. C	84. D	110. B	137. B
8. D	28. B	62. B	86. A	111. D	139. A
10. C	30. C	64. D	89. A	113. C	145. B
12. C	31. B	65. B	92. C	115. A	147. C
13. A	35. A	67. B	94. B	117. D	149. A
16. C	39. A	69. B	96. B	120. A	151. A
18. C	44. D	71. B	98. B	122. B	153. A
19. B	49. A	72. A	100. A	124. D	155. A
21. A	51. B	76. A	102. A	126. D	157. D
22. B	53. B	78. D	104. D	129. A	158. B
					160. C

Organization of TR/RT

2. A	33. D	74. D	99. A	123. C	144. D
4. C	36. C	77. C	114. C	130. B	146. C
11. D	38. C	87. A	116. C	133. C	148. C
14. B	45. B	91. D	118. D	136. A	152. D
26. C	46. C	97. C	121. D	141. B	154. A
					159. C

Advancement of the Profession

17. C	32. B	42. C	55. D	125. C	138. C
20. A	37. D	48. C	57. A	127. D	143. B
					150. A

Record Your Scores Here

Foundational Knowledge   _____ / 43 = _____ %
Practice of TR/RT   _____ / 73 = _____ %
Organization of TR/RT   _____ / 31 = _____ %
Advancement of the Profession   _____ / 13 = _____ %

Total Score = _____ /160

Total Percent = _____ %

chapter 6

Practice Test 1

This practice test represents the kind of items you will find on the NCTRC Certification Exam. The purpose of the practice test is to give you some indication of what it will feel like to take the actual NCTRC exam. The length of the test, and the content and format of the questions is close to that of the national test. The 90 items are also in the same proportion as the actual exam, in each of the categories of the Exam Content Outline. See Chapters 2 and 4 for more details about the proportion of items across the four categories of the Exam Content Outline. Additional practice tests follow.

Directions: For each question in this section, select the best of the answer choices given. Use the answer sheet on pages 88-89 to record your answers. Use the scoring key on page 90 to score your answers. If you complete the additional practice tests, compare your percentages of correct items in each of the four categories of content. This will give you some idea on which areas you are scoring better and which areas need more work.

1. According to Maslow, all humans are striving to achieve_____but first must fulfill other essential needs.
   (A) self-actualization
   (B) ego esteem needs
   (C) a sense of love and belonging
   (D) safety/security

2. A CTRS is interested in determining behaviors that relate to a person's ability to successfully integrate into society using his/her social interaction skills. From the following options, the CTRS should choose which assessment?
   (A) Leisure Diagnostic Battery (LDB)
   (B) Leisurescope
   (C) BANDI-RT
   (D) Comprehensive Evaluation in Recreational Therapy Scale (CERT) - Psych

3. Which one of the four categories of child development does the skill "heeds his/her name" belong?
   (A) Personal/social
   (B) Adaptive/fine motor behavior
   (C) Motor behavior
   (D) Language

4. The Global Assessment of Functioning (GAF) is a numeric scale used by clinicians and physicians in what type of setting?
   (A) Long-term care
   (B) Physical rehabilitation
   (C) Mental health
   (D) Pediatric heath care

5. A CTRS is looking for program ideas for adolescent chemical abusers. The BEST resource for the CTRS is
   (A) the *Therapeutic Recreation Journal*
   (B) state recreation conferences
   (C) chemical dependence conference
   (D) other therapeutic recreation professionals who work in chemical dependency

6. In order for charting-by-exception to be effective, what first must be accomplished?
   (A) Standards of care must be predefined so exceptions can be identified
   (B) The patient must be medically stable and coherent
   (C) Reimbursement for services has to be standardized hospital-wide
   (D) All health care professions must agree to a single-page assessment form

7. Which of the following examples typify the theory of self-efficacy?
    (A) The client believes he is efficient in most leisure activities
    (B) The client believes her life would change completely if she could live by herself
    (C) The client hates to lose so tries extremely hard to excel so he can win
    (D) The client believes he can master kayaking since he excels at canoeing

8. Most video games use which of the following social interaction patterns?
    (A) Intragroup
    (B) Multilateral
    (C) Interindividual
    (D) Extraindividual

9. Understanding facial expressions, customs, appropriate dress and the like are important considerations for improving a CTRS's
    (A) performance reviews
    (B) scope of practice
    (C) clinical supervision
    (D) cultural competence

10. Which of the following is NOT a rule for activity modification?
    (A) Keep the activity and action as close as possible to the original or traditional activity as possible
    (B) Modify only aspects of the activity that need adapting
    (C) Individualize the modifications
    (D) Use assistive technology wherever possible to ease the physical requirements of the activity

11. Neurological functions necessary for survival (e.g., breathing, digestion, heart rate) are located in what section of the brain?
    (A) Brainstem
    (B) Cerebellum
    (C) Frontal lobe
    (D) Occipital lobe

12. The term "branding" in marketing and public relations means that
    (A) a product or service is differentiated from other similar products or services
    (B) all company trademarks are copyrighted
    (C) a company focuses on the one product or service that sells best
    (D) all employees are responsible for 'selling' the product or service

13. A baby born with fetal alcohol syndrome will most likely have which of the following symptoms or characteristics?
    (A) Intellectual disability, facial abnormalities, and stunted growth
    (B) Enlarged heart, chemical tolerance, and bowed legs
    (C) Stunted growth, heart disease, and short stature
    (D) Facial abnormalities, tendency to weep, and stunted growth

14. After the client assessment has been completed, the next step in the programming process is to
    (A) write treatment summaries
    (B) analyze activities
    (C) identify the problem(s)
    (D) develop goals and objectives

15. The anatomical term "carpal" refers to which area of the body?
    (A) Abdominal cavity
    (B) Wrist
    (C) Thigh
    (D) Buttocks

16. Educating others about a particular issue on behalf of another person is called
    (A) education for all
    (B) advocacy
    (C) wellness promotion
    (D) attitude adjustment

17. Which of the following is a likely secondary condition to osteoporosis?
    (A) Muscle wasting
    (B) Hip fracture
    (C) Osteoarthritis
    (D) Hypertension

18. Using a holistic approach to therapeutic recreation services means that the CTRS
    (A) provides integrated services based in the community
    (B) addresses social, physical, cognitive, and emotional functioning in leisure
    (C) is part of a transdisciplinary treatment team
    (D) uses activity analysis to assess the characteristics of leisure activities

19. In the *Diagnostic and Statistical Manual of Mental Disorders (DSM-IV-TR)*, the diagnosis of depression would be categorized under
(A) Axis I
(B) Axis II
(C) Axis III
(D) Axis IV

20. Which of the following is an appropriate area for assessing affective functioning?
(A) Dual communication skills
(B) Safety awareness
(C) Emotional regulation
(D) Leisure attitudes

21. A CTRS is most likely to teach which of the following skill sets to individuals with panic disorders?
(A) Relaxation
(B) Cognitive dissonance
(C) Reality orientation
(D) Sensory stimulation

22. A CTRS wants to assess a patient's/client's ability to control anger. The CTRS should assess behavior from which of the following domains?
(A) Cognitive
(B) Physical
(C) Emotional
(D) Social

23. The two most widely used, evidence-based treatments for post-traumatic stress disorder are
(A) therapeutic exposure and cognitive reframing
(B) biofeedback and dream analysis
(C) escalation and progressive muscle relaxation
(D) modeling and stress management

24. In 1953, what organization was formed to identify and resolve different philosophies held by members of the Hospital Recreation Society, the Recreation Therapy Section, and the National Association of Recreation Therapists?
(A) Council for the Advancement of Hospital Recreation (CAHR)
(B) American Therapeutic Recreation Association (ATRA)
(C) National Therapeutic Recreation Society (NTRS)
(D) American Association of Recreational Therapy (AART)

25. Which of the following is a FALSE statement about self-efficacy?
(A) People are born with or without self-efficacy and it rarely changes during one's life course.
(B) Self-efficacy involves one's perceptions about his or her capabilities to attain a goal.
(C) As a person gains mastery in one area, self-efficacy may spread to other areas as well.
(D) To improve self-efficacy, it is better to start with simpler, smaller tasks that can be more readily accomplished.

26. Which of the examples below illustrates using the principles of evidence-based research in therapeutic recreation?
(A) The CTRS uses results from a *Therapeutic Recreation Journal* article to most efficiently create a stress management program.
(B) The CTRS collects evidence over 12 months to show the attendance rates of clients.
(C) The CTRS attends a research forum at a national conference.
(D) The CTRS calls colleagues to see how their aquatic programs are designed.

27. The purpose of the conjunctiva in the human eye is to
(A) provide color to the iris
(B) sense and react to light
(C) refract light as it enters the eye
(D) protect the eye from irritants

28. A client holds two opposing beliefs; one is that work is the most important thing in life and the second is that most enjoyment comes from leisure activities. Because this client feels this is a problem, the CTRS might employ which of the following intervention techniques with this client?
(A) Values clarification
(B) Reality orientation
(C) Remotivation
(D) Cognitive restructuring

29. Society generally devalues individuals with disabilities, reinforcing negative attitudes by doing all of the following EXCEPT
(A) using offensive terminology with regard to people with disabilities
(B) treating them as helpless and victimized
(C) labeling them as social burdens
(D) treating them as equals

30. Two clients ran away during a community outing. After contacting the police, the CTRS completes which form?
    (A) Incident report
    (B) Revised treatment plan
    (C) Discharge/referral summary
    (D) Liability summary

31. All of the following would be considered leisure constraints EXCEPT
    (A) freedom of choice
    (B) lack of leisure partners
    (C) inability to make decisions
    (D) fear of stigma

32. Which of the following is an example of using "displacement" as a defense mechanism?
    (A) Not remembering that the event occurred
    (B) Attributing the action or behavior to another person
    (C) Using a subordinate as the scapegoat
    (D) Not acknowledging the magnitude of a stressful event

33. Presbyopia is a visual condition common in older individuals that results in
    (A) loss of elasticity of the lens and inability to focus on an object
    (B) an astigmatism of unequal portions
    (C) cataracts
    (D) glaucoma

34. Which type of facility has the highest bed occupancy rate of all long-term facilities?
    (A) Nursing homes
    (B) State facilities for individuals with developmental disabilities
    (C) Psychiatric hospitals
    (D) Physical medicine and rehabilitation centers

35. In which of the following steps does the CTRS collect feedback for the improvement of future programs?
    (A) Assessment
    (B) Program planning
    (C) Program implementation
    (D) Program evaluation

36. In the Leisure Ability Model, the purpose of functional intervention services is to
    (A) provide co-treatment with other therapies at the most basic, functional levels
    (B) acquaint clients with available and appropriate community services
    (C) bring clients up to the baseline of their peers' average functional level
    (D) increase the physical capabilities of clients

37. A strategic plan is a method of
    (A) projecting needs and activities of an organization in the future
    (B) continuous quality improvement
    (C) protocol development and implementation
    (D) resource utilization

38. Which of the following sets of standards was established by the field of therapeutic recreation to address the quality of service delivery?
    (A) Accreditation standards
    (B) Certification standards
    (C) Education standards
    (D) Standards of practice

39. CTRSs and activity personnel typically complete which section of the MDS 3.0 assessment?
    (A) Section A Functional Abilities and Wellness
    (B) Section C Activity Interests and Participation
    (C) Section F Preferences for Customary Routine and Activities
    (D) Section K Activities of Daily Living and Leisure Experiences

40. A disability that is present at birth is described as
    (A) congenital
    (B) adventitious
    (C) traumatic
    (D) acquired

41. What is likely to happen if the assessment instrument is NOT administered in a reliable way to clients?
    (A) Client placement into programs will likely be wrong
    (B) Clients will improve their functional abilities more quickly
    (C) The activity analysis will yield faulty results
    (D) The client's length of stay will be reduced

42. Which of the following terms means that medication has been delivered directly to the spinal column?
    (A) Intravenously
    (B) Intramuscularly
    (C) Subcutaneously
    (D) Intrathecally

43. Reliability, as a measurement characteristic, asks which of the following questions?
    (A) Does the manual include directions for administering, scoring, and interpreting results?
    (B) Does the instrument match the programs offered to clients?
    (C) Does the instrument yield accurate information about the client?
    (D) Is the instrument measuring what it is intended to measure?

44. If the client does not understand the language used on the assessment or becomes fatigued, what is likely to happen?
    (A) The therapeutic recreation specialist will gain insight into the sitting tolerance of the client
    (B) The therapist still will be able to use the assessments from other disciplines to build a treatment plan
    (C) Nothing, most therapeutic recreation specialists do not use assessment scores anyway
    (D) The assessment score will not be reflective of the person's skills, attitudes, and knowledge

45. A CTRS selects the Comprehensive Evaluation in Recreational Therapy Scale (CERT-Psych) to measure behavior of a client as observed in group activities. Which assessment characteristic has the CTRS considered in making this selection?
    (A) Validity
    (B) Reliability
    (C) Usability
    (D) Practicability

46. Once the CTRS has met the sitting requirements for and passed the NCTRC exam, she must renew her certification every year and recertify every____year(s) to remain certified.
    (A) ten
    (B) five
    (C) six
    (D) two

47. The CTRS knew that by adhering to the assessment protocol she was
    (A) decreasing the content validity of the assessment results
    (B) increasing the likelihood of false positives
    (C) matching the content of the assessment with the content of the program
    (D) reducing error and increasing confidence in the assessment results

48. In 1983, a cost-cutting Medicare hospital payment system was initiated that included
    (A) a retrospective payment system
    (B) direct reimbursement for therapeutic recreation services
    (C) the Centers for Medicare and Medicaid Services (CMS)
    (D) diagnostic-related groups (DRGs)

49. The CTRS wants to assess clients for placement into a leisure education program. The CTRS should make sure the instrument is valid and measures which of the following?
    (A) Social skills, leisure activity skills, leisure resources, and leisure awareness
    (B) Functional limitations, social skills, and physical abilities
    (C) Leisure interests, functional limitations, leisure awareness, and leisure resources
    (D) Decision-making skills, small group and large group interaction skills, and leisure resources

50. The "saggital plane" divides the human body
    (A) with a horizontal line through the abdomen
    (B) from front to back
    (C) with a vertical line (left from right)
    (D) into four equal sections

51. A common secondary condition for individuals with visual impairments is
    (A) inability to memorize lists of words
    (B) obesity
    (C) impaired concentration skills
    (D) high cholesterol

52. Client documentation and program documentation are important because they allow for all of the following EXCEPT
    (A) increased communication among staff members
    (B) a higher degree of accountability
    (C) patient autonomy
    (D) adherence to professional and external standards

53. The medical term "NPO" is the abbreviation for
    (A) idiopathic diagnosis
    (B) nothing by mouth
    (C) normal parameters of oxygen
    (D) normal postoperative outpatient

54. Which of the following is typical behavior experienced during a manic episode for someone who has been diagnosed with bipolar disorder?
    (A) Ability to focus for long periods of time
    (B) Increased need for sleep and rest
    (C) Decreased sexual drive
    (D) Extreme irritability

55. Two CTRSs created agency-specific assessments on their own. One CTRS's assessment results in a score that then is used to place clients into therapeutic recreation programs, while the other CTRS's results in open-ended comments that are more difficult to analyze. The second CTRS's assessment will more likely result in
    (A) faulty program placement decisions and inability to show client outcomes
    (B) better validity of assessment results
    (C) better reliability of assessment results
    (D) improved ability to report accurate results to the treatment team

56. Which of the following is NOT a possible means of transmission of HIV?
    (A) Donating blood
    (B) Unprotected sexual intercourse
    (C) Sharing drug injection paraphernalia
    (D) Mother to fetus

57. Which of the following activities would most likely help an adolescent with an intellectual disability to improve concentration?
    (A) Watching television
    (B) Plant care
    (C) Crossword puzzle
    (D) Video game

58. Which of the following statements reflect the current emphasis of external accreditation agencies in reviewing therapeutic recreation services for quality improvement purposes?
    (A) The effectiveness of therapeutic recreation services is determined by the achieved client outcomes
    (B) The most important criteria for proving effectiveness of therapeutic recreation services is the availability of facilities and adequacy of equipment
    (C) The crucial element in therapeutic recreation quality assurance is the interaction established between the CTRS and the client
    (D) Linkages with community agencies is the prime factor in determining quality care in therapeutic recreation services

59. Given the goal statement below, which of the following is the most appropriate therapeutic recreation program?
    "Goal: To teach clients skills in negotiating physical environmental barriers"
    (A) Friday night bingo club
    (B) Big brother/big sister program
    (C) Leisure awareness discussion group
    (D) Wednesday night community re-integration trip to local mall

60. Visual deficits are the result of injury to what portion of the human brain?
    (A) Brainstem
    (B) Cerebellum
    (C) Frontal lobe
    (D) Occipital lobe

61. The major purpose of conducting an activity analysis is to make sure the selected activities
    (A) fit the program goals and client characteristics
    (B) are compatible with agency goals and staff abilities
    (C) are both social and physical in nature
    (D) are documented and evaluated on a timely basis

62. Health can be defined, not just as the absence of illness, but as
    (A) a higher level of disease process
    (B) exercising three days a week for at least 30 minutes at a time
    (C) a sense of physical, mental, and social well-being
    (D) minimal deviation from normal functioning

63. A CTRS is working with a group of adolescents who have mild intellectual disabilities and hopes to improve their interactions with each other. She has decided to use positive reinforcement for each good interaction that occurs with the group. The first thing the CTRS should do is
(A) determine how often the target behavior currently occurs
(B) determine what is a reinforcer
(C) reward each client whenever a good interaction occurs
(D) describe the target behavior

64. The medical/clinical model of healthcare
(A) involves total care of the individual, including sleeping, eating, and hygiene
(B) focuses on establishing a therapeutic community among clients
(C) centers on the physician as the primary decision-maker for client care
(D) provides services to clients often living independently

65. A common secondary condition for individuals with severe arthritis is
(A) spina bifida
(B) contractures
(C) enlarged bones
(D) aphasia

66. Which of the following is an example of a transdisciplinary treatment team?
(A) Each team member independently assesses and plans interventions for the client
(B) Each team member is responsible for collaborating with others on identifying common goal areas; then selects the best intervention within his or her discipline
(C) Each team member works across disciplinary boundaries to develop goals and plans, and often co-treats clients
(D) Each team member is cross-trained in each other's discipline and there are virtually no boundaries between disciplines

67. The federal agency that provides regulations to reduce workplace hazards and dangerous conditions is called the
(A) Occupational Safety and Health Administration
(B) Department of Health and Human Services
(C) Department of Homeland Security
(D) Employment and Job Site Security Bureau

68. What are the likely consequences of having inadequate resources and staff per activity?
(A) Risk to clients is increased
(B) The difficulty can be increased
(C) More content can be covered
(D) Less time is needed to reach targeted goals

69. The Current Procedural Terminology (CPT) codes created by the American Medical Association describe
(A) reimbursable intervention units
(B) recommendations for weekly physical activity
(C) protocols for the treatment of post-traumatic stress disorder
(D) risk management procedures used by most hospitals

70. In problem-oriented record keeping, the abbreviation SOAPIER stands for
(A) subjectivity, objectivity, assess, plan, implement, evaluate, revise
(B) subjective data, objective data, analysis, plan, interventions, evaluation, revisions
(C) sources, objects, adjectives, protocols, initiatives, expressions, resolutions
(D) nothing, it simply means to completely cover (saturate) the topic

71. Aging women, as compared to men, are cared for in long-term care facilities at the rate of
(A) 4 women to 3 men
(B) 10 women to 9 men
(C) 1 woman to 2 men
(D) 2 women to 1 man

72. If a person with osteoporosis engages in weight bearing activity that is too strenuous, he or she is put at higher risk for
(A) bone fracture
(B) contractures
(C) depression
(D) vestibular resistance

73. The CTRS documented how the client met her initial goals and objectives after two weeks. What form of documentation was the CTRS using?
(A) Assessment summary report
(B) Progress notes
(C) Transition summaries
(D) Discharge summaries

74. The CTRS works with an educator from a local university to research the impact of exercise on substance abuse patients in an outpatient recovery program. The CTRS is adhering to which principle of the *ATRA Code of Ethics*?
    (A) Confidentiality and privacy
    (B) Justice
    (C) Veracity
    (D) Competence

75. The CTRS teaches the client, who has been recently diagnosed with glaucoma, to make which of the following adaptations during activity involvement?
    (A) Use eye drops frequently
    (B) Periodically scan the entire area from side to side
    (C) Use a light background and dark print
    (D) Participate in activities only during the day or in areas with bright lights

76. The CTRS may need to describe specific behavioral cues that help describe the client's behavior. The client's _____ can be described using words such as lively, neutral, blunted, flat, stable, labile, defensive, calm, sad, hostile, guarded, distant, evasive, cooperative, and open.
    (A) speech
    (B) mood and affect
    (C) social distancing
    (D) movement

77. One of primary programming considerations for children with hearing impairments that should be included in the activity analysis of all therapeutic recreation activities is:
    (A) balance
    (B) atrophy
    (C) visual requirements
    (D) peripheral vision

78. Recreation participation programs are MOST appropriate for clients who need to
    (A) improve physical endurance
    (B) learn new leisure and recreation skills
    (C) practice social skills in an unstructured environment
    (D) become more aware of the role leisure plays in their lives

79. What is an advantage of asking open-ended questions of clients for a program evaluation?
    (A) The answers are easily quantifiable
    (B) The clients are able to expand on their answers.
    (C) The specialist needs to be skilled in interviewing people
    (D) There is no advantage to open-ended questions

80. Intellectual disability occurs in approximately what percent of the population in the US?
    (A) 1 percent
    (B) 10 percent
    (C) 20 percent
    (D) 30 percent

81. All of the following have an impact on how client documentation is recorded, EXCEPT
    (A) external accreditation standards
    (B) agency guidelines and procedures
    (C) legal requirements
    (D) activity analysis

82. All of the following documents should be evaluated and updated on a regular basis EXCEPT
    (A) job announcement
    (B) performance appraisal
    (C) job description
    (D) written plan of operation

83. Which of the following statements about leisure's impact on coping with stressful life events is TRUE?
    (A) Leisure activities often intensify the harmful effects of negative life events
    (B) Leisure activities often have the effect of eliminating optimism and hope about the future
    (C) Leisure activities often disrupt one's ability to cope with stress
    (D) Leisure activities may be used following negative life events to attain new goals

84. The CTRS checks each piece of recreation equipment each week during a routine maintenance and safety check. The CTRS is involved in what kind of action?
    (A) Client management
    (B) Quality achievement
    (C) Environmental assessment
    (D) Risk management

85. If the CTRS makes an error while writing in the client's chart, he should
    (A) use white correction fluid over the error and then write the correction in ink
    (B) report the mistake to his boss, and begin on a clean new page
    (C) cross out the error, write "error" above it and initial it
    (D) learn to always chart in pencil so mistakes can easily be erased and corrected

86. How often must an individual's Individualized Education Program be updated according to the Individuals with Disabilities Education Act of 2004?
    (A) Weekly
    (B) Quarterly
    (C) Semi-Annually
    (D) Annually

87. In systems program design, a performance measure (PM) is the same as a(n)
    (A) assessment item
    (B) outcome statement
    (C) enabling objective
    (D) mission statement

88. An adult with intellectual disability has the ability to participate in some general recreation programs within the regular community-based recreation program. When the CTRS helps the client enroll in one of these programs, which of the following mainstreaming principles is being applied?
    (A) Advocacy
    (B) Deinstitutionalization
    (C) Least restrictive environment
    (D) Discharge planning

89. Which of the following is NOT a factor in selecting an activity for client participation?
    (A) Activities must have a direct relationship to the client goal
    (B) Non-traditional activities make the intervention more fun for clients
    (C) A single activity or session is not likely to produce a desired behavioral change
    (D) Consider the types of activities in which people will engage when they have the choice

90. Activity analysis is the process of
    (A) examining client characteristics to best place them into programs
    (B) examining the activity components to identify inherent characteristics
    (C) evaluating the effects of the activities/programs on the clients
    (D) evaluating the resources/equipment needed to implement the activities

Practice Test 1

Scoring Sheet

1. Ⓐ Ⓑ Ⓒ Ⓓ   14. Ⓐ Ⓑ Ⓒ Ⓓ   27. Ⓐ Ⓑ Ⓒ Ⓓ   40. Ⓐ Ⓑ Ⓒ Ⓓ

2. Ⓐ Ⓑ Ⓒ Ⓓ   15. Ⓐ Ⓑ Ⓒ Ⓓ   28. Ⓐ Ⓑ Ⓒ Ⓓ   41. Ⓐ Ⓑ Ⓒ Ⓓ

3. Ⓐ Ⓑ Ⓒ Ⓓ   16. Ⓐ Ⓑ Ⓒ Ⓓ   29. Ⓐ Ⓑ Ⓒ Ⓓ   42. Ⓐ Ⓑ Ⓒ Ⓓ

4. Ⓐ Ⓑ Ⓒ Ⓓ   17. Ⓐ Ⓑ Ⓒ Ⓓ   30. Ⓐ Ⓑ Ⓒ Ⓓ   43. Ⓐ Ⓑ Ⓒ Ⓓ

5. Ⓐ Ⓑ Ⓒ Ⓓ   18. Ⓐ Ⓑ Ⓒ Ⓓ   31. Ⓐ Ⓑ Ⓒ Ⓓ   44. Ⓐ Ⓑ Ⓒ Ⓓ

6. Ⓐ Ⓑ Ⓒ Ⓓ   19. Ⓐ Ⓑ Ⓒ Ⓓ   32. Ⓐ Ⓑ Ⓒ Ⓓ   45. Ⓐ Ⓑ Ⓒ Ⓓ

7. Ⓐ Ⓑ Ⓒ Ⓓ   20. Ⓐ Ⓑ Ⓒ Ⓓ   33. Ⓐ Ⓑ Ⓒ Ⓓ   46. Ⓐ Ⓑ Ⓒ Ⓓ

8. Ⓐ Ⓑ Ⓒ Ⓓ   21. Ⓐ Ⓑ Ⓒ Ⓓ   34. Ⓐ Ⓑ Ⓒ Ⓓ   47. Ⓐ Ⓑ Ⓒ Ⓓ

9. Ⓐ Ⓑ Ⓒ Ⓓ   22. Ⓐ Ⓑ Ⓒ Ⓓ   35. Ⓐ Ⓑ Ⓒ Ⓓ   48. Ⓐ Ⓑ Ⓒ Ⓓ

10. Ⓐ Ⓑ Ⓒ Ⓓ   23. Ⓐ Ⓑ Ⓒ Ⓓ   36. Ⓐ Ⓑ Ⓒ Ⓓ   49. Ⓐ Ⓑ Ⓒ Ⓓ

11. Ⓐ Ⓑ Ⓒ Ⓓ   24. Ⓐ Ⓑ Ⓒ Ⓓ   37. Ⓐ Ⓑ Ⓒ Ⓓ   50. Ⓐ Ⓑ Ⓒ Ⓓ

12. Ⓐ Ⓑ Ⓒ Ⓓ   25. Ⓐ Ⓑ Ⓒ Ⓓ   38. Ⓐ Ⓑ Ⓒ Ⓓ   51. Ⓐ Ⓑ Ⓒ Ⓓ

13. Ⓐ Ⓑ Ⓒ Ⓓ   26. Ⓐ Ⓑ Ⓒ Ⓓ   39. Ⓐ Ⓑ Ⓒ Ⓓ   52. Ⓐ Ⓑ Ⓒ Ⓓ

53. Ⓐ Ⓑ Ⓒ Ⓓ   66. Ⓐ Ⓑ Ⓒ Ⓓ   79. Ⓐ Ⓑ Ⓒ Ⓓ

54. Ⓐ Ⓑ Ⓒ Ⓓ   67. Ⓐ Ⓑ Ⓒ Ⓓ   80. Ⓐ Ⓑ Ⓒ Ⓓ

55. Ⓐ Ⓑ Ⓒ Ⓓ   68. Ⓐ Ⓑ Ⓒ Ⓓ   81. Ⓐ Ⓑ Ⓒ Ⓓ

56. Ⓐ Ⓑ Ⓒ Ⓓ   69. Ⓐ Ⓑ Ⓒ Ⓓ   82. Ⓐ Ⓑ Ⓒ Ⓓ

57. Ⓐ Ⓑ Ⓒ Ⓓ   70. Ⓐ Ⓑ Ⓒ Ⓓ   83. Ⓐ Ⓑ Ⓒ Ⓓ

58. Ⓐ Ⓑ Ⓒ Ⓓ   71. Ⓐ Ⓑ Ⓒ Ⓓ   84. Ⓐ Ⓑ Ⓒ Ⓓ

59. Ⓐ Ⓑ Ⓒ Ⓓ   72. Ⓐ Ⓑ Ⓒ Ⓓ   85. Ⓐ Ⓑ Ⓒ Ⓓ

60. Ⓐ Ⓑ Ⓒ Ⓓ   73. Ⓐ Ⓑ Ⓒ Ⓓ   86. Ⓐ Ⓑ Ⓒ Ⓓ

61. Ⓐ Ⓑ Ⓒ Ⓓ   74. Ⓐ Ⓑ Ⓒ Ⓓ   87. Ⓐ Ⓑ Ⓒ Ⓓ

62. Ⓐ Ⓑ Ⓒ Ⓓ   75. Ⓐ Ⓑ Ⓒ Ⓓ   88. Ⓐ Ⓑ Ⓒ Ⓓ

63. Ⓐ Ⓑ Ⓒ Ⓓ   76. Ⓐ Ⓑ Ⓒ Ⓓ   89. Ⓐ Ⓑ Ⓒ Ⓓ

64. Ⓐ Ⓑ Ⓒ Ⓓ   77. Ⓐ Ⓑ Ⓒ Ⓓ   90. Ⓐ Ⓑ Ⓒ Ⓓ

65. Ⓐ Ⓑ Ⓒ Ⓓ   78. Ⓐ Ⓑ Ⓒ Ⓓ

Practice Test 1

Scoring Key

Foundational Knowledge

1. A	13. A	23. A	33. A	56. A	75. B
3. A	15. B	25. A	40. A	60. D	77. A
7. D	17. B	27. D	42. D	62. C	80. A
9. D	19. A	29. D	50. C	67. A	86. D
11. A	21. A	31. A	54. D	71. A	88. A

Practice of TR/RT

2. D	20. C	39. C	51. B	63. D	78. C
4. C	22. C	41. A	52. C	65. B	81. D
6. A	28. A	43. C	53. B	68. A	83. D
8. D	32. B	44. D	55. A	70. B	85. C
10. D	34. C	45. A	57. D	72. A	87. B
14. C	36. C	47. D	59. D	74. D	89. B
18. B	38. D	49. A	61. A	76. B	90. B

Organization of TR/RT

26. A	35. D	48. D	66. C	73. B	82. A
30. A	37. A	64. C	69. A	79. B	84. D

Advancement of the Profession

5. D	12. A	16. B	24. A	46. B	58. A

PRACTICE TEST 1

Record Your Scores Here

Foundational Knowledge	_____ / 30 =	_____ %
Practice of TR/RT	_____ / 42 =	_____ %
Organization of TR/RT	_____ / 12 =	_____ %
Advancement of the Profession	_____ / 6 =	_____ %

Total Score = _____ /90

Total Percent = _____ %

If you need more practice in any area(s), proceed to the next practice test.

chapter 7

Practice Test 2

This practice test represents the kind of items you will find on the NCTRC Certification Exam. The purpose of the practice test is to give you some indication of what it will feel like to take the actual NCTRC exam. The length of the test, and the content and format of the questions is close to that of the national test. The 90 items are also in the same proportion as the actual exam, in each of the categories of the Exam Content Outline. See Chapters 2 and 4 for more details about the proportion of items across the four categories of the Exam Content Outline. Additional practice tests follow.

Directions: For each question in this section, select the best of the answer choices given. Use the answer sheet on pages 100-101 to record your answers. Use the scoring key on page 102 to score your answers. If you complete the additional practice tests, compare your percentages of correct items in each of the four categories of content. This will give you some idea on which areas you are scoring better and which areas need more work.

1. Which one of the four categories of child development does the skill "sits leaning forward on hands" belong?
   (A) Personal/social
   (B) Adaptive/fine motor behavior
   (C) Motor behavior
   (D) Language

2. Which of the following is NOT a benefit resulting from completing an activity analysis?
   (A) a better comprehension of the client's activity interests and preferences
   (B) a rationale or explanation for the therapeutic benefits of activity involvement
   (C) information for selecting a leadership or facilitation technique
   (D) a greater understanding of the complexity of activity requirements for client participation

3. Which of the following is an example of clinical supervision?
   (A) Overseeing clients on a community out-trip
   (B) Overseeing clients during an in-house discussion group
   (C) Helping a junior professional become a better practitioner
   (D) Performing personnel evaluations on staff as least once per year

4. In 2001, the World Health Organization revamped its classification of human functioning and disablement. Called the International Classification of Functioning, Disability, and Health (ICF), it promotes
   (A) better medical care in third world countries
   (B) viewing human functioning and disablement from a biopyschosocial model of health
   (C) more active treatment for those with severe disabilities and terminal illnesses
   (D) therapeutic recreation as one of three services that promote quality of life

5. Many private hospitals followed the federal government in adhering to a prospective payment system. This means that
   (A) hospitals receive the same fee for each diagnostic-related group (DRG) they treat
   (B) insurance companies will pay whatever hospitals charge for a service
   (C) individuals pay 80 percent of health care charges
   (D) psychiatric services are available to individuals within their own community

6. Which is the most common adult social interaction pattern?
   (A) Intragroup
   (B) Multilateral
   (C) Interindividual
   (D) Extraindividual

7. Which of the following is a true statement about the aging process?
   (A) Individuals with less education tend to outlive those with more education
   (B) Women tend to outlive men
   (C) Ethnic minority members tend to outlive Caucasians
   (D) Individuals who are single tend to outlive those with families

8. Which of the following is the BEST example of a client outcome measure, collected as part of the therapeutic recreation department's quality improvement efforts?
   (A) Change in clients' health status or well-being
   (B) Change in client's attendance at programs
   (C) Development of a baseline for expected client behavior
   (D) Development of one-to-one treatment programs

9. An older female has been admitted as a client to a psychiatric facility for treatment of severe depression. She says her daughter has taken care of her home and needs for the last 5 years. She has no interest in making her own decisions about leisure involvement. The client may be exhibiting
   (A) learned helplessness
   (B) infantile expressive skills
   (C) extrinsic behavior
   (D) aggressive behavior

10. The difference between a vision statement and a statement of purpose for an organization is that a vision statement is
    (A) never put into operation
    (B) created solely by the top level managers
    (C) far-reaching and translates values into a desired future
    (D) is for the immediate future and is directly translated into operational goals

11. When an agency has decided to use the Functional Independence Measure (FIM), the CTRS may be called upon to assess which of the following sections?
    (A) Self-care
    (B) Mobility
    (C) Home skills
    (D) Social/cognition

12. When a person believes that his or her culture is superior to or better than other cultures, it is called
    (A) superiority complex
    (B) ethnocentrism
    (C) egotism
    (D) cultural delusion

13. The State Technical Institute's Leisure Assessment Process (STILAP) assessment differs from other activity inventories or leisure interest scales because it
    (A) focuses on physical activities such as sports and large group games
    (B) assesses barriers to community integration
    (C) looks at the entire community environment to which the client is to return
    (D) translates activity skills into leisure competencies

14. Which of the following is NOT a method for an active CTRS to be recertified by NCTRC?
    (A) Receiving a passing grade in university-level course work
    (B) Completing a second internship in a different setting
    (C) Attending professional workshops that award CEUs for participation
    (D) Writing and publishing educational articles in professional journals

15. Which of the following is NOT a characteristic of an effective group?
(A) Each person monitors someone else's progress toward accomplishing the task
(B) Have a unifying relationship
(C) Seek a shared and common goal
(D) Work together to meet individual and group needs

16. The CTRS wrote the following note in a client's chart. Which of the following documentation principles was violated?
"Mrs. Sullivan appeared to be lethargic and depressed."
(A) Add adequate descriptions to explain motivations
(B) Be consistent and explain exceptional behavior
(C) Observe behavior, then write it down
(D) Focus on client behavior, rather than interpretations of behavior

17. When individuals with disabilities are categorized and labeled (e.g., "the retarded," "the disabled"), it shows
(A) misconceptions about professionalism
(B) the underlying attitudes held toward individuals with disabilities
(C) inadequate information about health and illness
(D) religious beliefs toward perceived differences

18. Which of the following is an example of the condition part of a behavioral objective?
(A) With level 4 minimal assistance
(B) The client will plan a weekend trip
(C) After the completion of the program
(D) Two out of three times

19. Which of the following is NOT a true statement about the majority of individuals with intellectual disability?
(A) They are more easily suggestible than individuals with higher intelligence
(B) They are more passive in their thoughts than individuals with higher intelligence
(C) They are more judgmental than individuals with higher intelligence
(D) They are more concrete in their thinking than individuals with higher intelligence

20. The CTRS on a physical medicine and rehabilitation unit plans on providing a clinic on adapted tennis. Which of the following would NOT be a consideration for modifications?
(A) Available facilities
(B) Necessary equipment and materials needed
(C) Number of qualified staff
(D) Decision-making skills

21. Reimbursement for therapeutic recreation services is dependent on all of the following EXCEPT
(A) insurance contracts
(B) local managed care agreements
(C) the square footage of the activity area
(D) documentation of client outcomes

22. Which of the following is the BEST example of a receptive communication dysfunction?
(A) Inability to transform experiences into language
(B) Inability to comprehend the written or spoken word
(C) Inability to express oneself through actions or language
(D) Inability to distinguish regional accents in spoken language

23. A CTRS should use which of the following resources to find successful, proven methods of achieving positive client outcomes through actual therapeutic recreation services?
(A) *Therapeutic Recreation Journal*
(B) An introduction to therapeutic recreation textbook
(C) *Adapted Activities Quarterly*
(D) *ATRA Newsletter*

24. Which of the following terms means that medication has been delivered under the tongue?
(A) Sublingually
(B) Intramuscularly
(C) Subcutaneously
(D) Intrathecally

25. The CTRS is treating a divorced parent who has custody of two children. The lawyer of the non-custodial parent calls seeking information regarding the status of the custodial parent. The CTRS refuses to give information. The CTRS is adhering to which principle of the ATRA *Code of Ethics*?
(A) Confidentiality and privacy
(B) Justice
(C) Veracity
(D) Competence

26. For individuals with substance dependence problems, the term tolerance means that the person
    (A) needs more of the substance to achieve intoxication
    (B) is more open-minded and accepting of diverse opinions
    (C) shows emotional distress during substance withdrawal
    (D) willingly accepts more limitations within his/her life

27. Which of the following is the best approach to use with individuals who are kinesthetic learners?
    (A) Drawings on a chalkboard or white board
    (B) Verbal recordings of instructions
    (C) Materials that provide tactile stimulation
    (D) Charts, signs, and posters with clear instructions

28. High-quality patient documentation focuses on "behavioral language." Which of the following is NOT an example of a behavioral statement?
    (A) The client was 15 minutes late to the therapeutic recreation program
    (B) The client stated that she was bored during the social skills program
    (C) The patient verbalized her appreciation for therapeutic recreation services
    (D) The patient appeared distraught and upset

29. A CTRS is working with a person who is a quadriplegic as a result of a recent diving accident. The CTRS suggests that she try playing Ping-Pong instead of tennis, which she has previously enjoyed. The CTRS is using which of the following therapeutic recreation principles?
    (A) Aging-in-place
    (B) Substitutability
    (C) Least restrictive environment
    (D) Continuity of care

30. In Section O of the MDS 3.0, all of the following conditions must be present to be considered concurrent therapy EXCEPT
    (A) two or more residents are engaged in different tasks
    (B) the director of nursing must be present
    (C) the residents must be in direct line-of-sight of the therapist or assistant
    (D) student interns must be in direct line-of-sight of therapist, if providing treatment

31. Universal design of facilities means that the built environment is
    (A) usable to the greatest extent possible by everyone
    (B) free of stairways and curb cuts
    (C) available at those facilities which persons with disabilities frequent
    (D) specific to the age of the individuals who go there

32. A halfway house is used primarily for individuals who
    (A) need a balance of supervision and independence
    (B) are alcoholics
    (C) have intellectual disability
    (D) have been diagnosed for at least two years

33. The Family and Medical Leave Act (FMLA) provides which of the following for eligible employees?
    (A) Payment for adoption services for foreign-born child(ren)
    (B) Payment for funeral expenses for family members
    (C) Unpaid, job-protected leave for specified family and medical reasons
    (D) Six weeks of paid vacation per year

34. Given the goal statement below, which of the following is the most appropriate therapeutic recreation program?
    "Goal: To provide opportunities for self-expression"
    (A) Open gym for volleyball practice
    (B) Outdoor bocce ball game
    (C) Open time in the woodworking room
    (D) Art instruction in quilting

35. The term "muscular strength" refers to
    (A) repeated submaximal effort
    (B) the range of motion within a joint
    (C) the ability to change direction without losing balance
    (D) a single maximum effort

36. On an activity analysis form, the items about interaction patterns (such as uni-lateral, intra-individual, etc.) would best fit under the component of:
    (A) physical
    (B) mental
    (C) emotional
    (D) social

37. Which of the following is NOT a requirement of the Health Insurance Portability and Accountability Act (HIPAA) of 1996 and later rules?
    (A) Give patients notice about how their health information will be used
    (B) Make a good faith effort to ensure patients understand their rights
    (C) Obtain written authorization from the patient for purposes other than treatment, payment, or operations
    (D) Perform research on evidence-based and best practice health care

38. Validity, as a measurement characteristic, asks which of the following questions?
    (A) Is the instrument measuring what it is intended to measure?
    (B) Will the same results happen if the instrument is given a second time?
    (C) Does the manual include directions for administering, scoring and interpreting results?
    (D) How consistent are the results from one client to another?

39. Which of the following is an example of an interpersonal constraint to leisure participation?
    (A) Lack of self-determination of the individual
    (B) Lack of interest in the activities being offered
    (C) Lack of transportation to recreation facilities and programs
    (D) Lack of leisure partners

40. Which of the following is NOT an example of inclusive recreation programming?
    (A) Community reintegration programs for outpatients
    (B) Leisure skills instruction for independent participation
    (C) Ensuring universal design in leisure facilities and programs
    (D) Anger management training for inpatients with substance addictions

41. Glaucoma is the result of excessive pressure build-up within the
    (A) aqueous humor of the anterior chamber of the eye
    (B) synovial joint of the neck
    (C) tympanic membrane in the ear
    (D) Eustachian tube

42. According to the Leisure Ability model of therapeutic recreation services, the program service categories include
    (A) functional intervention, leisure education, and recreation participation services
    (B) therapy and recreation services
    (C) leisure education, counseling, and recreation services
    (D) inpatient, outpatient, and community services

43. Three early professional organizations for TR (HRS, NART & RTS) formed the National Council for the Advancement of Hospital Recreation (CAHR). What was the major accomplishment of CAHR in 1956?
    (A) A combined professional philosophy for the entire field
    (B) The creation of the National Voluntary Registration Plan for TR Personnel
    (C) The creation of the National Therapeutic Recreation Society
    (D) The first standards of practice for TR practitioners

44. The content of the assessment must match the content of the
    (A) activity analysis
    (B) program
    (C) treatment plan
    (D) quality improvement plan

45. An individual with a moderate hearing impairment would MOST likely need which of the following services or adaptations?
    (A) Community mobility training
    (B) Well-lit rooms with bright colors
    (C) Amplification devices in some situations
    (D) Personal assistants to take care of daily needs

46. One of the problems with client assessment in therapeutic recreation services is that
    (A) there are too many assessments from which to select
    (B) clients are too diverse to be assessed
    (C) assessments that are validated for practice are difficult to find and use
    (D) the information they gather is often in conflict with that of other treatment team members

47. When choosing an assessment instrument, the CTRS first needs to determine the instrument's
    (A) reliability
    (B) validity
    (C) stability
    (D) purpose

48. The custodial/long-term care model of healthcare
    (A) involves total care of the individual, including sleeping, eating, and hygiene
    (B) focuses on establishing a therapeutic community among clients
    (C) centers on the physician as the primary decision-maker for client care
    (D) provides services to clients often living independently

49. Muscular dystrophy results in which of the following activity limitations?
    (A) loss of muscle function
    (B) decrease in hand-eye coordination
    (C) decrease in attention span
    (D) improved respiration and resting heart rate

50. The CTRS wants to start a walking program for clients who meet the criteria for entering the program. With which of the following disciplines is the CTRS most likely to collaborate on the treatment team?
    (A) Personal trainer
    (B) Occupational therapy
    (C) Physical therapy
    (D) Outpatient therapy coordinator

51. Almost all models of therapeutic recreation service delivery start with the step of
    (A) assessment
    (B) goal development
    (C) program evaluation
    (D) quality improvement

52. Within the Individuals with Disabilities Education Act of 2004, and updated in 2011, Part C now includes individuals with
    (A) developmental delays aged 2 and under
    (B) autism spectrum disorder, including Asperger's Syndrome
    (C) mental illnesses as long as they are in school
    (D) traumatic brain injury, regardless of age

53. One mistake in assessment many CTRSs make is to
    (A) improve the reliability of their assessment instrument
    (B) use the results of the assessment to place clients into programs
    (C) use an assessment that was intended for a different purpose
    (D) interview clients asking the questions in the same way every time

54. Which method of behavioral observation and recording is the CTRS using when she records how long a certain behavior lasts?
    (A) Frequency or tally
    (B) Duration
    (C) Interval
    (D) Instantaneous time sampling

55. Which of the following questions would NOT be appropriate when documenting a client's participation in a therapeutic recreation program?
    (A) Did the client attend voluntarily?
    (B) Did the client merely observe the activity?
    (C) Was the client actively participating in the session?
    (D) Did the client attend all therapies on Tuesday?

56. Dementia typically results in which of the following activity limitations?
    (A) decrease in amount of aphasia
    (B) increased likelihood of blood disorders
    (C) memory loss
    (D) increase in executive functioning

57. A person who has a hearing capacity of less than 120 decibels (db) is considered to
    (A) have normal hearing
    (B) be slightly hearing impaired
    (C) be moderately hearing impaired
    (D) be deaf

58. The medical term "VO" is the abbreviation for
    (A) verbal order
    (B) halitosis
    (C) ventilator only
    (D) vital organism

59. Which one of the following components is missing from the discharge summary?
    "Pt. was referred to TR program due to lack of appropriate social skills at peer level and complaints of boredom. Pt. participated in Social Skills Training programs on a weekly basis and Leisure Opportunities programs on a daily basis for 5 weeks. Pt. enrolled in 2 community-based leisure programs. CTRS will follow-up in 3 weeks to monitor client progress in community."
    (A) Major client goals or problems
    (B) Services received by the client
    (C) Client attainment of goals
    (D) Plans for post-discharge involvement

60. Which of the following are NOT typical characteristics of someone who has been diagnosed with schizophrenia?
(A) Thought disorder
(B) Dysmorphia
(C) Blunted or flat affect
(D) Social withdrawal

61. In this excerpt of a client's treatment plan, which of the following, if any, was MOST likely identified as the client's problems?
1. "Enroll pt. in Leisure Planning class Tuesdays and Thursdays. Focus on taking responsibility and decision-making.
2. Enroll pt. in Social Singles Club weekly. Focus on initiating and maintaining conversations with peers."
(A) A lack of knowledge of leisure resources and lack of social partners
(B) A lack of conversational abilities and decreased concentration skills
(C) A lack of repertoire of activity skills and inability to identify leisure value system
(D) None of the above

62. The condition called Phenylketonuria is associated with
(A) schizophrenia
(B) cerebral vascular accident
(C) barbiturate addiction
(D) intellectual disability

63. The CTRS places a client in a team sport to introduce cognitive challenges. What higher level intellectual requirement is needed to be successful in a team sport like soccer?
(A) Memorization of rules
(B) Coordination of body parts
(C) Concentration
(D) Application of strategies

64. If an individual experiences a stroke on the right side of his/her brain, the typical effects include
(A) lack of depth perception, intuition, and non-verbal perception
(B) inability to remember past events and to read
(C) inability to communicate and organize thoughts
(D) increased lability and anger control

65. When a physician or case manager creates a master list of client deficits and develops a plan of action focused on these deficits, this is called
(A) a problem-oriented medical record
(B) a clinical pathway
(C) the case load of the physician on staff
(D) a diagnostic protocol

66. The CTRS wants to develop a stress management program. He first reviews the *Therapeutic Recreation Journal*, the *Annual in Therapeutic Recreation*, and the *American Journal of Recreation Therapy* to determine what is known about the design and effects of stress management programs in therapeutic recreation so he can apply that information to build the program he provides clients. The CTRS is performing what task?
(A) A field review
(B) A research study
(C) Evidence-based practice
(D) A meta-analysis

67. In which of the four domains does the statement below fall under?
"To wait to interrupt until appropriate conversational opportunity occurs"
(A) Cognitive
(B) Affective
(C) Physical
(D) Social

68. Which of the following are examples of secondary conditions?
(A) Osteoporosis and hip fracture
(B) Spinal cord injury and heart disease
(C) Dementia and losing track of time
(D) Arthritis and scoliosis

69. In which of the four domains does the statement below fall under?
"To improve ability to locate facilities on a map."
(A) Cognitive
(B) Affective
(C) Physical
(D) Social

70. Which of the following is an appropriate goal for a client who lacks awareness of personal resources?
    (A) The client will identify four assets within himself/herself that complement her leisure lifestyle.
    (B) The client will name three leisure resources in the community.
    (C) The client will learn three new leisure activities within the next three months.
    (D) The client will register for one community program within one month.

71. Neuroleptics are a class of prescription medications for which of the following disorders?
    (A) Agoraphobia
    (B) Tardive dyskinesia
    (C) Schizophrenia
    (D) Neuropathy

72. In the United States, which of the following is among the most participated in?
    (A) Basketball
    (B) Swimming
    (C) Inline skating
    (D) Bowling

73. In using a service marketing approach to promoting her community-based program, the CTRS focuses on which of the following?
    (A) Relationships to clients
    (B) The price point for programs provided
    (C) Quality of the programs provided
    (D) The staff that provide services

74. When a person experiences stress, which of the following physiological reactions occur?
    (A) Blood pressure lowers
    (B) Pupils (eyes) become dilated
    (C) Respirations decrease
    (D) Blood rushes to the hands and feet

75. The top two leading causes of death in the United States are
    (A) obesity and strokes
    (B) heart disease and cancer
    (C) heart disease and sexually-transmitted diseases
    (D) vehicular accidents and gunshot wounds

76. The client's goal is to develop appropriate competitive skills. The CTRS selects table games like checkers and tic tac toe to initiate intervention. At what social interaction level has the CTRS begun intervention?
    (A) Extra individual
    (B) Aggregate
    (C) Inter-individual
    (D) Unilateral

77. In which of the following steps does the CTRS use modalities and facilitation techniques to improve the delivery of programs?
    (A) Assessment
    (B) Program planning
    (C) Program implementation
    (D) Program evaluation

78. Which of the following is a TRUE statement about alcoholism?
    (A) More males than females are diagnosed with alcoholism
    (B) Onset is usually in a person's mid-to late-twenties
    (C) Alcoholism is genetically inherited from grandparents
    (D) Mortality and morbidity rates are lower for individuals with alcoholism

79. A client receives a token every time he responds appropriately to a request from a staff member. This approach is called
    (A) behavior management
    (B) behavior modification
    (C) behavior therapy
    (D) milieu therapy

80. The program evaluation is designed at the same time the program is planned so that the
    (A) CTRS will know how and when to collect information as the program progresses
    (B) client will know from the activity calendar when activities are offered
    (C) treatment team can collect information about the continuity of care
    (D) activities are analyzed for their physical, social/affective, and intellectual requirements of clients

81. Which of the following is an example of having an internal locus of control?
    (A) The client is motivated to participate to receive approval from the staff
    (B) After a game, prizes are given out randomly
    (C) The client wants to improve her artistic ability
    (D) The clients look forward to receiving prizes after bingo

82. Which of the following is a FALSE statement about implementing therapeutic recreation programs for clients?
    (A) The CTRS should know several different facilitation techniques in order to select the most appropriate one for a particular group
    (B) The facilitation technique selected by the specialist depends upon the abilities, limitations and needs of the clients
    (C) Each client will vary in the amount he/she may benefit from a particular type of facilitation technique
    (D) There is no research to support the use of facilitation techniques in therapeutic recreation

83. Which of the following is a TRUE statement about autonomic hyperreflexia (autonomic dysreflexia)?
    (A) It is often felt as an "aura" before the experience of a seizure
    (B) Common in people with spinal cord injuries, it is a rapid and uncontrolled elevation in blood pressure
    (C) It is common among individuals who have chronic schizophrenia and can be controlled through medication
    (D) It is associated with excessive dopamine in the limbic brain center and eventually causes death

84. Which set of standards governs the delivery of programs and services in the profession regardless of setting or population?
    (A) Critical pathways
    (B) Code of ethics
    (C) Plan of operations
    (D) Standards of practice

85. Which of the following is the best test for agility?
    (A) A timed obstacle course
    (B) Repetitious weight lifting
    (C) Chin ups
    (D) Core strength training

86. The CTRS works in a youth correctional facility. At the beginning and ending of each session, he counts the number of scissors and rulers to make sure that all recreation supplies are accounted for. The CTRS is involved in what kind of action?
    (A) Equipment management
    (B) Risk management
    (C) Environmental assessment
    (D) Quality achievement

87. In the Therapeutic Recreation Outcome Model, the purpose of therapeutic recreation is to
    (A) provide diversional leisure activities for enjoyment and entertainment
    (B) plan and implement community inclusion services under the ADA
    (C) improve the client's leisure lifestyle
    (D) improve the client's quality of life by increasing functional capacity and health status

88. Facilities that provide adult day care, assisted living, behavioral health, and employment and community services are MOST LIKELY to seek accreditation from
    (A) Joint Commission (JCAHO)
    (B) National Committee for Quality Assurance (NCQA)
    (C) Centers for Medicare and Medicaid Services (CMS)
    (D) Rehabilitation Accreditation Commission (CARF)

89. What role does a good assessment play in providing intervention programs to clients?
    (A) It ensures that clients are placed in the right programs for their needs
    (B) It shows the client what his/her leisure interests are
    (C) It provides feedback to the therapist about how well the program is going
    (D) It is the basis for quality improvement

90. If the client assessment cannot distinguish between those who need the program and those who do not, what is likely to happen to the clients?
    (A) They are likely to receive the wrong program, a diversional program, or no program at all
    (B) They will receive both functional intervention and leisure education programs
    (C) They are more likely to benefit from community integration programs
    (D) They are more likely to efficiently reach their outcomes and achieve an early discharge

Practice Test 2

Scoring Sheet

1. Ⓐ Ⓑ Ⓒ Ⓓ   14. Ⓐ Ⓑ Ⓒ Ⓓ   27. Ⓐ Ⓑ Ⓒ Ⓓ   40. Ⓐ Ⓑ Ⓒ Ⓓ

2. Ⓐ Ⓑ Ⓒ Ⓓ   15. Ⓐ Ⓑ Ⓒ Ⓓ   28. Ⓐ Ⓑ Ⓒ Ⓓ   41. Ⓐ Ⓑ Ⓒ Ⓓ

3. Ⓐ Ⓑ Ⓒ Ⓓ   16. Ⓐ Ⓑ Ⓒ Ⓓ   29. Ⓐ Ⓑ Ⓒ Ⓓ   42. Ⓐ Ⓑ Ⓒ Ⓓ

4. Ⓐ Ⓑ Ⓒ Ⓓ   17. Ⓐ Ⓑ Ⓒ Ⓓ   30. Ⓐ Ⓑ Ⓒ Ⓓ   43. Ⓐ Ⓑ Ⓒ Ⓓ

5. Ⓐ Ⓑ Ⓒ Ⓓ   18. Ⓐ Ⓑ Ⓒ Ⓓ   31. Ⓐ Ⓑ Ⓒ Ⓓ   44. Ⓐ Ⓑ Ⓒ Ⓓ

6. Ⓐ Ⓑ Ⓒ Ⓓ   19. Ⓐ Ⓑ Ⓒ Ⓓ   32. Ⓐ Ⓑ Ⓒ Ⓓ   45. Ⓐ Ⓑ Ⓒ Ⓓ

7. Ⓐ Ⓑ Ⓒ Ⓓ   20. Ⓐ Ⓑ Ⓒ Ⓓ   33. Ⓐ Ⓑ Ⓒ Ⓓ   46. Ⓐ Ⓑ Ⓒ Ⓓ

8. Ⓐ Ⓑ Ⓒ Ⓓ   21. Ⓐ Ⓑ Ⓒ Ⓓ   34. Ⓐ Ⓑ Ⓒ Ⓓ   47. Ⓐ Ⓑ Ⓒ Ⓓ

9. Ⓐ Ⓑ Ⓒ Ⓓ   22. Ⓐ Ⓑ Ⓒ Ⓓ   35. Ⓐ Ⓑ Ⓒ Ⓓ   48. Ⓐ Ⓑ Ⓒ Ⓓ

10. Ⓐ Ⓑ Ⓒ Ⓓ   23. Ⓐ Ⓑ Ⓒ Ⓓ   36. Ⓐ Ⓑ Ⓒ Ⓓ   49. Ⓐ Ⓑ Ⓒ Ⓓ

11. Ⓐ Ⓑ Ⓒ Ⓓ   24. Ⓐ Ⓑ Ⓒ Ⓓ   37. Ⓐ Ⓑ Ⓒ Ⓓ   50. Ⓐ Ⓑ Ⓒ Ⓓ

12. Ⓐ Ⓑ Ⓒ Ⓓ   25. Ⓐ Ⓑ Ⓒ Ⓓ   38. Ⓐ Ⓑ Ⓒ Ⓓ   51. Ⓐ Ⓑ Ⓒ Ⓓ

13. Ⓐ Ⓑ Ⓒ Ⓓ   26. Ⓐ Ⓑ Ⓒ Ⓓ   39. Ⓐ Ⓑ Ⓒ Ⓓ   52. Ⓐ Ⓑ Ⓒ Ⓓ

53. Ⓐ Ⓑ Ⓒ Ⓓ   66. Ⓐ Ⓑ Ⓒ Ⓓ   79. Ⓐ Ⓑ Ⓒ Ⓓ

54. Ⓐ Ⓑ Ⓒ Ⓓ   67. Ⓐ Ⓑ Ⓒ Ⓓ   80. Ⓐ Ⓑ Ⓒ Ⓓ

55. Ⓐ Ⓑ Ⓒ Ⓓ   68. Ⓐ Ⓑ Ⓒ Ⓓ   81. Ⓐ Ⓑ Ⓒ Ⓓ

56. Ⓐ Ⓑ Ⓒ Ⓓ   69. Ⓐ Ⓑ Ⓒ Ⓓ   82. Ⓐ Ⓑ Ⓒ Ⓓ

57. Ⓐ Ⓑ Ⓒ Ⓓ   70. Ⓐ Ⓑ Ⓒ Ⓓ   83. Ⓐ Ⓑ Ⓒ Ⓓ

58. Ⓐ Ⓑ Ⓒ Ⓓ   71. Ⓐ Ⓑ Ⓒ Ⓓ   84. Ⓐ Ⓑ Ⓒ Ⓓ

59. Ⓐ Ⓑ Ⓒ Ⓓ   72. Ⓐ Ⓑ Ⓒ Ⓓ   85. Ⓐ Ⓑ Ⓒ Ⓓ

60. Ⓐ Ⓑ Ⓒ Ⓓ   73. Ⓐ Ⓑ Ⓒ Ⓓ   86. Ⓐ Ⓑ Ⓒ Ⓓ

61. Ⓐ Ⓑ Ⓒ Ⓓ   74. Ⓐ Ⓑ Ⓒ Ⓓ   87. Ⓐ Ⓑ Ⓒ Ⓓ

62. Ⓐ Ⓑ Ⓒ Ⓓ   75. Ⓐ Ⓑ Ⓒ Ⓓ   88. Ⓐ Ⓑ Ⓒ Ⓓ

63. Ⓐ Ⓑ Ⓒ Ⓓ   76. Ⓐ Ⓑ Ⓒ Ⓓ   89. Ⓐ Ⓑ Ⓒ Ⓓ

64. Ⓐ Ⓑ Ⓒ Ⓓ   77. Ⓐ Ⓑ Ⓒ Ⓓ   90. Ⓐ Ⓑ Ⓒ Ⓓ

65. Ⓐ Ⓑ Ⓒ Ⓓ   78. Ⓐ Ⓑ Ⓒ Ⓓ

Practice Test 2

Scoring Key

Foundational Knowledge

1. C	15. A	26. A	39. D	60. B	75. B
4. B	17. B	29. B	41. A	62. D	78. A
7. B	19. C	31. A	45. C	64. A	81. C
9. A	22. B	33. C	52. A	68. A	83. B
12. B	24. A	35. D	57. D	71. C	85. A

Practice of TR/RT

2. A	25. A	40. D	53. C	63. D	76. C
6. A	27. C	42. A	54. B	65. A	79. B
11. D	30. B	44. B	55. D	67. D	82. D
13. D	32. A	46. C	56. C	69. A	84. D
16. D	34. C	47. D	58. A	70. A	87. D
18. C	36. D	49. A	59. C	72. D	89. A
20. D	38. A	51. A	61. D	74. B	90. A

Organization of TR/RT

3. C	8. A	21. C	48. A	66. C	80. A
5. A	10. C	28. D	50. C	77. C	86. B

Advancement of the Profession

14. B	23. A	37. D	43. B	73. C	88. D

PRACTICE TEST 2

Record Your Scores Here

Foundational Knowledge	_____ / 30 =	_____ %
Practice of TR/RT	_____ / 42 =	_____ %
Organization of TR/RT	_____ / 12 =	_____ %
Advancement of the Profession	_____ / 6 =	_____ %

Total Score = _____ /90

Total Percent = _____ %

If you need more practice in any area(s), proceed to the next practice test.

chapter 8

Practice Test 3

This practice test represents the kind of items you will find on the NCTRC Certification Exam. The purpose of the practice test is to give you some indication of what it will feel like to take the actual NCTRC exam. The length of the test, and the content and format of the questions is close to that of the national test. The 90 items are also in the same proportion as the actual exam, in each of the categories of the Exam Content Outline. See Chapters 2 and 4 for more details about the proportion of items across the four categories of the Exam Content Outline. Additional practice tests follow.

Directions: For each question in this section, select the best of the answer choices given. Use the answer sheet on pages 112-113 to record your answers. Use the scoring key on page 114 to score your answers. If you complete the additional practice tests, compare your percentages of correct items in each of the four categories of content. This will give you some idea on which areas you are scoring better and which areas need more work.

1. The primary role of CTRSs working with individuals who have autism is to
   (A) have them learn a variety of leisure skills that their peers might know
   (B) improve their visual acuity
   (C) teach them how to adapt activities on their own
   (D) improve their ADLs

2. Which of the following is an example of a self-fulfilling prophecy?
   (A) The client enjoyed every minute of the self-awareness activity
   (B) The client felt great joy at helping other people, especially older adults
   (C) The client fails to score a point, just as he predicted earlier
   (D) The client always knew she wanted to be a therapeutic recreation specialist

3. One of the MOST important aspects of a client/therapist relationship is for the CTRS to
   (A) have an unconditional positive regard for the client
   (B) let the client know he/she is always right
   (C) establish a position of authority with the client
   (D) establish a relationship with the client's family

4. The CTRS wants to starts a garden group that clients can independently attend and organize. The best group format would be
   (A) Instructional class
   (B) Clubs and special interest groups
   (C) Drop-in center
   (D) Out-trips

5. Which of the following organizations allows for chapter affiliation by local groups of therapeutic recreation specialists?
(A) National Therapeutic Recreation Society (NTRS)
(B) American Therapeutic Recreation Association (ATRA)
(C) Recreation Therapy Section (RTS)
(D) National Council for Therapeutic Recreation Certification (NCTRC)

6. Which of the following is an example of extinction that is meant to reduce a specific behavior?
(A) Taking a client to the zoo when they are afraid of animals
(B) Taking away a favorite toy when the client misbehaves
(C) Talking to the client about antecedents, behaviors, and consequences
(D) Applying the principle of negative reinforcement

7. The CTRS was offered free tickets for patients to attend a special performance of a play during the afternoon, but instead chose to have the patients/clients pay and attend a night performance. The CTRS was demonstrating which of the following mainstreaming principles?
(A) Integration
(B) Normalization
(C) Least restrictive environment
(D) Deinstitutionalization

8. The CTRS is working with a group of chemically dependent teenagers. The goal of the program is "To gain an understanding of the importance of leisure." The CTRS decides to use an activity called "Twenty Things I Love To Do." This is an example of
(A) reality therapy
(B) assertiveness
(C) values clarification
(D) bibliotherapy

9. A person who had a brain injury and now has problems speaking is considered to have
(A) autism
(B) an aneurysm
(C) aphasia
(D) an occlusion

10. The CTRS on a mental health unit plans on providing instruction on coping skills for clients. Which of the following would NOT be a consideration?
(A) Number of participants
(B) Types of equipment and materials needed
(C) Increase in behavioral prompts
(D) Level of social interaction skills

11. Alzheimer's type dementia is caused by
(A) biological changes in the brain
(B) getting older
(C) not engaging in intellectual activities as one ages
(D) environmental pollutants and toxins

12. A client outcome is the
(A) client's heightened awareness of leisure as a substitute for work
(B) observed changes in the client's status as a result of interventions
(C) end result of an activity analysis
(D) point at which activity analysis and client assessment intersect

13. Children with visual or hearing impairments are often found to have significantly reduced _____ in comparison with their seeing or hearing peers.
(A) intelligence
(B) parental supervision
(C) academic achievement
(D) physical fitness

14. Which of the following are typical parts of a client treatment plan?
(A) Assessment results, goals and objectives, interventions, and reevaluation schedule
(B) Client deficits, statements, behaviors, and plans for change
(C) Current status, past status, and future status
(D) Strengths, plan of action, and discharge plan

15. Paralysis on one side of the body is called
(A) paraplegia
(B) hemiplegia
(C) monoplegia
(D) quadriplegia

16. ATRA's *Standards for the Practice of Therapeutic Recreation* document is divided into two sections of
    (A) assessment and program planning
    (B) clinical and community guidelines
    (C) direct practice and management
    (D) inpatient and outpatient care

17. The CTRS sends in forms reporting participation in continuing education activities to NCTRC every five years. The CTRS is adhering to which principle of the *ATRA Code of Ethics*?
    (A) Confidentiality and privacy
    (B) Justice
    (C) Veracity
    (D) Competence

18. The dividing vertebrae between being classified as a paraplegic and a quadriplegic is
    (A) C8, T1
    (B) T12, L1
    (C) T1, T2
    (D) T5, T6

19. In promoting their long-term care facility, the CTRS suggested her management team capitalize on the bond and affinity that current residents have with staff. The CTRS is promoting which kind of marketing?
    (A) Product marketing
    (B) Services marketing
    (C) Relationship marketing
    (D) Public relations

20. Which of the following medications is classified as an adjuvant?
    (A) Elavil
    (B) Demerol
    (C) Percodan
    (D) Feldeme

21. Which of the following is the most difficult of all documentation methods to easily interpret and extrapolate information from?
    (A) Problem-oriented records
    (B) Focus charting
    (C) Narrative records
    (D) SOAP notes

22. In a facility that uses the Health Protection/Health Promotion model of therapeutic recreation, what would be the intent of service delivery?
    (A) Helping clients become more competent and able to select enjoyable activities
    (B) Helping people overcome barriers to health that interfere with their leisure
    (C) Promoting human happiness through primary and secondary efforts
    (D) Empowering the client to achieve only those goals that improve their leisure lifestyle

23. The major components of the Optimizing Lifelong Health through Therapeutic Recreation service delivery model are
    (A) diagnosis/assessment, treatment, education, and prevention/health promotion
    (B) functional intervention, leisure education, and recreation participation
    (C) prescriptive activities, recreation, and leisure
    (D) selecting, optimizing, compensating, and evaluating

24. Which question is the BEST formative evaluation concern?
    (A) How does the second day of the program need to be changed from the first day?
    (B) Are the interventions appropriate for the content?
    (C) What were the total resource costs of program delivery?
    (D) Was staff adequately prepared to deliver the services to this group of clients?

25. Which method of behavioral observation and recording is the CTRS using when she checks the activity room at 9:00, 11:00, 1:00 and 3:00 to see how many patients are watching television?
    (A) Frequency or tally
    (B) Duration
    (C) Interval
    (D) Instantaneous time sampling

26. Clients are most likely to achieve an optimal experience when
    (A) the activity challenge and their skill level are nearly equal
    (B) they are trying a novel activity
    (C) the activity is similar to what they have experienced before
    (D) stress is low and challenge is high

27. Which method of behavioral observation and recording is the CTRS using when he wants to know how many times the client attends therapeutic recreation programs?
(A) Frequency or tally
(B) Duration
(C) Interval
(D) Instantaneous time sampling

28. The Americans with Disabilities Act of 1990 allows full and equal access by persons with disabilities to
(A) any place of public accommodation
(B) state and federal buildings funded through public taxes
(C) almost any public accommodation, but excludes recreation facilities
(D) any recreation facility, whether public, private, or commercial

29. Which of the following is NOT requirement of the Health Insurance Portability and Accountability Act (HIPAA) of 1996 and later rules?
(A) Enforce policies and procedures to protect patient information
(B) Designate a person to oversee adherence to the rules
(C) Allow children to make health care decisions for themselves
(D) Secure patient records to that a minimal number of people have access

30. All of the following things affect people's attitudes toward individuals with disabilities, EXCEPT
(A) characters portrayed in movies
(B) fairy tales and childhood stories
(C) etiological concerns
(D) television advertisements

31. The CTRS wants to apply the principles of Arousal, Novelty, and Diversity in her plan for a leisure skills instruction program. Which of the following is she most likely to incorporate?
(A) Relating the content to the participants' lives
(B) Fading prompts as participants gain skills
(C) Allowing time for repetition and practice
(D) Offering a variety of activities and materials within the program

32. Which of the following may be an effect of having a spinal cord injury on a person's leisure lifestyle?
(A) The person will have ill health and not be physically active.
(B) The person's range of leisure options will be larger than average.
(C) The person's range of activities may be limited by physical accessibility.
(D) The person will be able to maximize choice and be self-determined.

33. Which of the following recreation activities is the best treatment modality for improving social skills?
(A) Bingo with prizes
(B) Aquatic therapy
(C) Yoga instruction
(D) Cooperative games

34. In which of the following steps does the CTRS examine how the content and process of the activity will contribute to the accomplishment of client objectives?
(A) Assessment
(B) Program planning
(C) Program implementation
(D) Program Evaluation

35. Units or facilities that are especially designed for individuals with moderate to advanced dementia include which of the following design considerations?
(A) Mazes for wandering, bright colors, no signage, heavy security doors
(B) Minimal clutter, no more than 10 residents per unit, one large bedroom for all 10
(C) Clusters of residences, meaningful wandering path, positive and secure outdoor space
(D) Walking paths through the community, well-lit areas, large activity spaces

36. The discrepancy between the mental age (MA) and the chronological age (CA) for persons with intellectual disability
(A) becomes less noticeable with age
(B) becomes more noticeable with age
(C) influences the quality of the materials used in recreation equipment
(D) determines the facility to be used

37. One of the primary criteria for selecting client assessments for use in therapeutic recreation programs is that
(A) the content of the assessment matches the content of the intervention program
(B) it improves the expertise of the specialist
(C) the inter-rater reliability is high
(D) it requires specialized training just for therapeutic recreation specialists

38. All of the following are important ways to ensure that the assessment results translates into the right program placement to work on a client's identified problems, EXCEPT
(A) use an assessment that produces reliable scores for the intended population
(B) train all CTRSs and interns on the correct use of the assessment
(C) document a standardized protocol for the administration, scoring, and interpretation of the assessment
(D) improve the construct validity of the assessment instrument

39. A CTRS may work with a person who has recently experienced an extensive thermal burn, by providing which of the following types of sessions?
(A) Leisure resource utlization
(B) Adjustment to disability
(C) Leisure awareness
(D) Assistive devices and adaptive techniques

40. Which of the following is NOT a purpose of community reintegration programs?
(A) To go to more theaters and other public venues
(B) To reduce stigma associated with a disability
(C) To practice in a real-world setting the skills that have been learned in treatment
(D) To gain familiarity with community resources

41. Which of the following provides example behaviors from an individual with oppositional defiant behavior?
(A) Extreme levels of hyperactivity and distractibility
(B) Interruptive social behaviors that are more apparent to others than the individual
(C) Behaviors that violate the rights of others and major age-appropriate societal norms
(D) Negative, hostile behaviors toward others

42. What effect has clients' shortened lengths of stay had on client assessment?
(A) It is now a much easier task because clients are more focused on their own treatment
(B) The connection between gathering a baseline of information and measuring for outcomes has been strengthened
(C) Assessments need to be concise and administered more quickly following admission
(D) The effect has been minimal because therapeutic recreation specialists have always been known for efficient assessments

43. Older adults often need an extended rest period following physical exertion because they
(A) are less motivated to continue to exercise
(B) require longer to return to a state of homeostasis after an activity
(C) fail to properly warm up prior to the exercise
(D) tend to overexert during physical activities

44. Which of the following is a FALSE statement about the disadvantages of unstructured interviews?
(A) Individual CTRS in the department may not use the same questions
(B) There is too much room for interpretation that limits reliability
(C) They increase reliability at the expense of validity
(D) They are too difficult to score consistently

45. Consider the following two interview questions/statements to be used in a client assessment.
1 "Tell me how you would go about finding transportation to get to an athletic event downtown. "
2 "Tell me about your family."
Interview question/statement 1 is better than 2, because it
(A) focuses on the specific content of therapeutic recreation programs
(B) requires less short-memory from the client
(C) requires less time for the client to answer
(D) takes more time to analyze and interpret the answer for placement into programs

46. The first major textbooks with the term "therapeutic recreation" in the titles were published in the:
(A) 1890s
(B) 1910s
(C) 1940s
(D) 1970s

47. When intervention sessions are planned, what are the primary factors to consider?
    (A) The time constraints of the therapists and support staff
    (B) The number of clients served on the unit and space available
    (C) The case load and grand rounds of the physician on staff
    (D) The patient's needs and nature of the program

48. A CTRS in a correctional institution may emphasize programming based on improving the individual's self-efficacy in coping with high-risk situations that may trigger re-incarceration. An example of a program title suited for this purpose is
    (A) Relapse Prevention Strategies
    (B) Total Body Workout
    (C) Competitive Volleyball
    (D) Bibliotherapy

49. Medicare is a federal health insurance program that does NOT include which of the following?
    (A) Individuals who are first- or second-generation Native Americans
    (B) Individuals 65 or older
    (C) Individuals under age 65 with certain disabilities
    (D) Individuals with end-stage renal disease

50. One of the most common conditions associated with myasthenia gravis is
    (A) gout
    (B) high blood sugar
    (C) muscle contractures in elbows and knees
    (D) drooping eyelids

51. Muscular dystrophy advances from proximal to distal in the extremities, meaning that
    (A) jumping is one of the last skills to be lost
    (B) hand and finger function remains intact longer
    (C) the person loses muscle from front to back
    (D) the person loses muscle from feet to head

52. Which of the following is the most difficult interpersonal constraint for a CTRS to overcome?
    (A) lack of free activities in the community
    (B) Lack of accessible facilities
    (C) Lack of participant skill
    (D) Lack of participant interest

53. Given the goal statement below, which of the following is the most appropriate therapeutic recreation program?
    "Goal: To increase clients' dyad cooperation skills"
    (A) Volleyball instruction clinic
    (B) Backgammon tournament
    (C) Leisure resource information exchange group
    (D) Ballroom dancing instruction

54. In implementing an exercise program for aging individuals, the CTRS becomes aware that the planned activity is too strenuous for the participants. The CTRS inadequately analyzed the _____ requirements of the activity for the given population.
    (A) social
    (B) emotional
    (C) physical
    (D) cognitive

55. When a hospital or health care agency receives accreditation from the Joint Commission (JCAHO) among other things, it means
    (A) the hospital will receive Medicare payments more easily
    (B) professionals working in the agency will get direct reimbursement for services
    (C) the client will receive a lower quality of care
    (D) client assessment must be completed with 12 hours of admission

56. The CTRS uses the Information Seeking and Health Spectrum Model to develop therapeutic recreation programs for persons who utilize outpatient services at a physical medicine and rehabilitation center. She provides information to clients that is related to
    (A) adaptations and modifications for leisure participation
    (B) prevention of substance addictions
    (C) improvement of short-term and long-term memory
    (D) optimal arousal and focus

57. In long-term care, skilled nursing units or facilities means that the patients have
    (A) medical needs that require an additional amount of nursing or other therapies
    (B) federal or private insurance coverage
    (C) contagious conditions that threaten the general public
    (D) multiple conditions, often called poly-trauma

58. A CTRS is responsible for administering the MDS 3.0 to her residents. She knows the first step is to
    (A) determine whether the resident can indicate a preference
    (B) discuss the residents' needs with the interdisciplinary treatment team
    (C) assess the resident's leisure preferences and interests
    (D) create a variety of activities of interest to the residents

59. The therapeutic milieu model of healthcare
    (A) involves total care of the individual, including sleeping, eating, and hygiene
    (B) focuses on establishing a therapeutic community among clients
    (C) centers on the physician as the primary decision-maker for client care
    (D) provides services to clients often living independently

60. Teenscope is a useful assessment to place adolescent clients into which types of therapeutic recreation programs?
    (A) Treatment
    (B) Social skills
    (C) Leisure resources
    (D) Leisure skills

61. According to the National Institutes of Health, which condition occurs more frequently than diabetes, heart disease, and cancer combined?
    (A) macular degeneration
    (B) osteoarthritis
    (C) brain concussions
    (D) pain

62. The overall content covered by the Leisure Diagnostic Battery (LDB) includes
    (A) leisure participation history
    (B) leisure interests
    (C) attitudes toward leisure and work
    (D) perceived freedom in leisure

63. Chronic pain has been characterized as pain that
    (A) results from surgical or medical procedures
    (B) cannot be reduced with medications
    (C) cannot be reduced through meditation
    (D) is prolonged and persistent

64. In medical terminology, NKDA means
    (A) no known diagnostic algorithms
    (B) sodium phosphate
    (C) above knee amputation
    (D) no known drug allergies

65. In which of the four domains does the following statement fall under?
    "To express anger in a positive manner"
    (A) Cognitive
    (B) Affective
    (C) Physical
    (D) Social

66. The CTRS will most likely to work with which of the following disciplines to provide medical play to hospitalized children?
    (A) Physical therapy
    (B) Occupational therapy
    (C) Nursing
    (D) Child life

67. When the physician or treatment team creates a master list of patient/client deficits and develops a plan of action focused on these deficits, it is called which of the following?
    (A) Problem-oriented medical records (POMR)
    (B) Source-oriented medical records (SOMR)
    (C) Client deficit planning
    (D) Quality improvement

68. The process by which an agency of the government grants permission to persons meeting predetermined qualification to engage in a given occupation is called _____.
    (A) licensure
    (B) accreditation
    (C) certification
    (D) registration

69. Which of the following is the BEST method of reducing the likelihood of decubitus ulcers?
    (A) Drinking plenty of fluids
    (B) Using stool softeners
    (C) Yoga and other stretching exercises
    (D) Change in positioning

70. In a treatment protocol, the outcome criteria refers to
    (A) measurable changes brought about in a patient as a direct result of the intervention
    (B) how the assessment is conducted
    (C) the timing of the treatment evaluation
    (D) steps taken and services provided by the CTRS to complete the protocol

71. Which social interaction pattern focuses on action with an object in the environment, requiring no contact with another person?
    (A) Intragroup
    (B) Multilateral
    (C) Interindividual
    (D) Extraindividual

72. Chronic users of cocaine may experience all of the following, EXCEPT
    (A) depression
    (B) periods of excessive sleep
    (C) hypertension
    (D) respiratory and/or cardiac failure

73. What is likely to happen when the content of the assessment does not match the content of the programs designed for client participation?
    (A) The assessment is likely to be more valid than reliable
    (B) The assessment will not lead to proper program placement and clients will not reach their goals
    (C) Outcomes will be better defined and less ambiguous
    (D) The assessment will have less cultural bias and increased sensitivity

74. An individual who has a panic disorder experiences
    (A) maladaptive behaviors in response to social situations
    (B) persistent, abnormally intense fears
    (C) "free-floating" anxiety which tends to pervade all areas of life
    (D) sudden, periodic attacks of intense anxiety

75. The CTRS knew that she could not program for and measure outcomes for self-esteem, but she still wanted to program in this area and have clients achieve measurable outcomes. What outcomes would be more appropriate than "improve self-esteem?"
    (A) Improve self-concept
    (B) Verbalize two positive statements about self
    (C) Decrease negative thoughts about self
    (D) Increase self-image

76. After each out-trip the CTRS is required to perform an 11-point checklist on the van. What is the purpose of this task?
    (A) Vehicle registration inspection
    (B) Quality improvement
    (C) Vehicle evaluation
    (D) Risk management

77. All of the following may be questions that the CTRS uses to improve clarity and completeness to a narrative note EXCEPT
    (A) How did I first become aware of the problem?
    (B) What has the client said about the problem that is not significant?
    (C) Is this the same problem that was exhibited last week?
    (D) What is the plan for dealing with the problem?

78. According to the World Health Organization's International Classification of Functioning, Disability, and Health (ICF), services are needed at each of the following levels
    (A) Community, state, regional, and national
    (B) Body part, the whole person, and the person's social context
    (C) Medical, rehabilitation, and long-term care
    (D) Functional intervention, leisure education, and recreation participation

79. In a therapeutic recreation program accredited by Joint Commission (JCAHO), the goal would be to
    (A) improve health care quality and patient safety
    (B) improve baseline, functional abilities of all clients
    C) discharge all clients to their own homes/communities
    (D) reduce errors and improve confidence

80. Which of the following is NOT an example of a chronic health condition?
    (A) Heart disease
    (B) Diabetes mellitus
    (C) High blood pressure
    (D) Vehicular accident

81. There are how many vertebrae in the cervical region of the human spine?
    (A) 3
    (B) 5
    (C) 7
    (D) 9

82. Which of the following may be used as a technique to motivate employees on a long-term basis?
    (A) Make them boss for the day
    (B) Ask them to do more with fewer resources
    (C) Encourage their donations to the agency's charity fund
    (D) Encourage cross training into new areas of job responsibility

83. While a medical model of health care focuses on the pathology of a person, the salutogenic model of health focuses on
    (A) lifestyle factors that support, enhance, and produce health
    (B) social relationships that need to be terminated prior to full recovery
    (C) total lifestyle environment to which the patient will return
    (D) direct reimbursement of services

84. The medical term "qid" is the abbreviation for
    (A) white blood count
    (B) four times a day
    (C) quadriceps
    (D) within normal limits

85. Which one of the four categories of child development does the skill "asks why" belong?
    (A) Personal/social
    (B) Adaptive/fine motor behavior
    (C) Motor behavior
    (D) Language

86. Which part of the SOAP progress note is the following statement, "Schedule pt. for social interaction program?"
    (A) S – Subjective
    (B) O – Objective
    (C) A- Assessment
    (D) P – Plan

87. The Centers for Medicare and Medicaid Services (CMS) is the governmental agency responsible for
    (A) building collaborative initiatives between private and public hospitals
    (B) ensuring that patients within these programs pay their bills in a timely manner
    (C) reporting medical errors to the American Medical Association
    (D) regulatory review of hospitals that bill for federally insured recipients

88. Operant conditioning is a form of learning that stems from which type of psychology?
    (A) Behavioristic
    (B) Humanistic
    (C) Instrumental
    (D) Psychoanalytic

89. The CTRS manager submitted a report to the executive director, that the activity room had a leak in the ceiling that was causing the floor tiles to ripple and be uneven. The CTRS was practicing risk management with regard to
    (A) facilities
    (B) equipment
    (C) clients
    (D) staff

90. Which of the following represents the highest level of cross-cultural competence?
    (A) Being aware that one is lacking knowledge about another culture
    (B) Learning about clients' cultures and providing culturally specific interventions
    (C) Automatically providing culturally congruent care to clients of diverse cultures
    (D) Not being aware that one is lacking knowledge about another culture

Practice Test 3

Scoring Sheet

1. Ⓐ Ⓑ Ⓒ Ⓓ   14. Ⓐ Ⓑ Ⓒ Ⓓ   27. Ⓐ Ⓑ Ⓒ Ⓓ   40. Ⓐ Ⓑ Ⓒ Ⓓ

2. Ⓐ Ⓑ Ⓒ Ⓓ   15. Ⓐ Ⓑ Ⓒ Ⓓ   28. Ⓐ Ⓑ Ⓒ Ⓓ   41. Ⓐ Ⓑ Ⓒ Ⓓ

3. Ⓐ Ⓑ Ⓒ Ⓓ   16. Ⓐ Ⓑ Ⓒ Ⓓ   29. Ⓐ Ⓑ Ⓒ Ⓓ   42. Ⓐ Ⓑ Ⓒ Ⓓ

4. Ⓐ Ⓑ Ⓒ Ⓓ   17. Ⓐ Ⓑ Ⓒ Ⓓ   30. Ⓐ Ⓑ Ⓒ Ⓓ   43. Ⓐ Ⓑ Ⓒ Ⓓ

5. Ⓐ Ⓑ Ⓒ Ⓓ   18. Ⓐ Ⓑ Ⓒ Ⓓ   31. Ⓐ Ⓑ Ⓒ Ⓓ   44. Ⓐ Ⓑ Ⓒ Ⓓ

6. Ⓐ Ⓑ Ⓒ Ⓓ   19. Ⓐ Ⓑ Ⓒ Ⓓ   32. Ⓐ Ⓑ Ⓒ Ⓓ   45. Ⓐ Ⓑ Ⓒ Ⓓ

7. Ⓐ Ⓑ Ⓒ Ⓓ   20. Ⓐ Ⓑ Ⓒ Ⓓ   33. Ⓐ Ⓑ Ⓒ Ⓓ   46. Ⓐ Ⓑ Ⓒ Ⓓ

8. Ⓐ Ⓑ Ⓒ Ⓓ   21. Ⓐ Ⓑ Ⓒ Ⓓ   34. Ⓐ Ⓑ Ⓒ Ⓓ   47. Ⓐ Ⓑ Ⓒ Ⓓ

9. Ⓐ Ⓑ Ⓒ Ⓓ   22. Ⓐ Ⓑ Ⓒ Ⓓ   35. Ⓐ Ⓑ Ⓒ Ⓓ   48. Ⓐ Ⓑ Ⓒ Ⓓ

10. Ⓐ Ⓑ Ⓒ Ⓓ   23. Ⓐ Ⓑ Ⓒ Ⓓ   36. Ⓐ Ⓑ Ⓒ Ⓓ   49. Ⓐ Ⓑ Ⓒ Ⓓ

11. Ⓐ Ⓑ Ⓒ Ⓓ   24. Ⓐ Ⓑ Ⓒ Ⓓ   37. Ⓐ Ⓑ Ⓒ Ⓓ   50. Ⓐ Ⓑ Ⓒ Ⓓ

12. Ⓐ Ⓑ Ⓒ Ⓓ   25. Ⓐ Ⓑ Ⓒ Ⓓ   38. Ⓐ Ⓑ Ⓒ Ⓓ   51. Ⓐ Ⓑ Ⓒ Ⓓ

13. Ⓐ Ⓑ Ⓒ Ⓓ   26. Ⓐ Ⓑ Ⓒ Ⓓ   39. Ⓐ Ⓑ Ⓒ Ⓓ   52. Ⓐ Ⓑ Ⓒ Ⓓ

53. (A) (B) (C) (D)   66. (A) (B) (C) (D)   79. (A) (B) (C) (D)

54. (A) (B) (C) (D)   67. (A) (B) (C) (D)   80. (A) (B) (C) (D)

55. (A) (B) (C) (D)   68. (A) (B) (C) (D)   81. (A) (B) (C) (D)

56. (A) (B) (C) (D)   69. (A) (B) (C) (D)   82. (A) (B) (C) (D)

57. (A) (B) (C) (D)   70. (A) (B) (C) (D)   83. (A) (B) (C) (D)

58. (A) (B) (C) (D)   71. (A) (B) (C) (D)   84. (A) (B) (C) (D)

59. (A) (B) (C) (D)   72. (A) (B) (C) (D)   85. (A) (B) (C) (D)

60. (A) (B) (C) (D)   73. (A) (B) (C) (D)   86. (A) (B) (C) (D)

61. (A) (B) (C) (D)   74. (A) (B) (C) (D)   87. (A) (B) (C) (D)

62. (A) (B) (C) (D)   75. (A) (B) (C) (D)   88. (A) (B) (C) (D)

63. (A) (B) (C) (D)   76. (A) (B) (C) (D)   89. (A) (B) (C) (D)

64. (A) (B) (C) (D)   77. (A) (B) (C) (D)   90. (A) (B) (C) (D)

65. (A) (B) (C) (D)   78. (A) (B) (C) (D)

Practice Test 3

Scoring Key

Foundational Knowledge

2. C	13. D	28. A	41. D	63. D	81. C
4. B	15. B	30. C	43. B	72. B	83. A
7. B	18. C	32. C	49. A	74. D	85. D
9. C	20. A	36. B	52. D	78. B	88. A
11. A	26. A	39. B	61. D	80. D	90. C

Practice of TR/RT

1. A	16. C	33. D	45. A	56. A	69. D
3. A	17. D	35. C	47. D	58. A	71. D
6. B	22. B	37. A	48. A	60. D	73. B
8. C	23. D	38. D	50. D	62. D	75. B
10. C	25. D	40. A	51. B	64. D	77. B
12. B	27. A	42. C	53. D	65. B	84. B
14. A	31. D	44. C	54. C	67. A	86. D

Organization of TR/RT

21. C	34. B	59. B	70. A	79. A	87. D
24. A	57. A	66. D	76. D	82. D	89. A

Advancement of the Profession

5. B	19. C	29. C	46. D	55. A	68. A

PRACTICE TEST 3

Record Your Scores Here

Foundational Knowledge   _____ / 30 = _____ %
Practice of TR/RT   _____ / 42 = _____ %
Organization of TR/RT   _____ / 12 = _____ %
Advancement of the Profession   _____ / 6 = _____ %

Total Score = _____ /90
Total Percent = _____ %

If you need more practice in any area(s), proceed to the next practice test.

chapter 9

Practice Test 4

This practice test represents the kind of items you will find on the NCTRC Certification Exam. The purpose of the practice test is to give you some indication of what it will feel like to take the actual NCTRC exam. The length of the test, and the content and format of the questions is close to that of the national test. The 90 items are also in the same proportion as the actual exam, in each of the categories of the Exam Content Outline. See Chapters 2 and 4 for more details about the proportion of items across the four categories of the Exam Content Outline. Additional practice tests follow.

Directions: For each question in this section, select the best of the answer choices given. Use the answer sheet on pages 124-125 to record your answers. Use the scoring key on page 126 to score your answers. If you complete the additional practice tests, compare your percentages of correct items in each of the four categories of content. This will give you some idea on which areas you are scoring better and which areas need more work.

1. Which one of the four categories of child development does the skill "plays simple nursery games" belong?
   (A) Personal/social
   (B) Adaptive/fine motor behavior
   (C) Motor behavior
   (D) Language

2. When using active listening with a client, it is important for the CTRS to do which of the following?
   (A) Reflect the feeling tone the client communicates
   (B) Respond immediately to the client's statements
   (C) Nod his/her head and speak to the client frequently
   (D) Ask questions so the client will know the CTRS is listening

3. Which of the following is the BEST example of an efficacy research study conducted in a physical rehabilitation setting?
   (A) Client skills at discharge are compared with their skills at admission
   (B) The CTRS tracks client attendance at therapeutic recreation programs
   (C) Two CTRSs evaluate the inter-rater reliability of their observational assessment tool
   (D) Peer reviews are conducted on adherence to *ATRA Standards of Practice*

4. Which of the following statements is TRUE about the following objective?
   "When given a choice of three activities, the client will verbalize his favorite leisure activity to participate with friends."
   (A) The condition is missing
   (B) The behavior is missing
   (C) The criterion is missing
   (D) The objective is complete as is

5. In medical terminology, MVA means
   (A) more ventricular reaction
   (B) military vehicle accident
   (C) major ventricular arteries
   (D) motor vehicle accident

6. In which of the following steps does the CTRS gather data for service quality improvement?
   (A) Assessment
   (B) Program laning
   (C) Program implementation
   (D) Program evaluation

7. From assessment results, the CTRS determines that the client has a lack of knowledge of community leisure facilities and programs, and is unaware of other people who participate in her leisure interests. Which of the following therapeutic recreation programs would be the MOST appropriate for this client?
    (A) Leisure planning
    (B) Social skills training
    (C) Leisure values and attitudes
    (D) Leisure resources

8. The following is an example of which one of the following health care delivery systems?
    This model is based on the philosophy that mental illness is the product of unhealthy interactions with one's environment.
    (A) Medical
    (B) Custodial
    (C) Milieu
    (D) Education and Training

9. Most facilities utilize treatment teams in order to
    (A) provide better documentation of services
    (B) receive community support for programs
    (C) shorten the client's length of stay at the facility
    (D) bill clients at a higher rate

10. The CTRS wants to create an activity area that clients can come to and complete their own art projects, work on puzzles, or have conversations with others. The best program format would be
    (A) Instructional class
    (B) Clubs and special interest groups
    (C) Drop-in center
    (D) Out-trips

11. Which of the following would improve the reliability of the results of an assessment tool?
    (A) Replace all closed-ended items with open-ended items
    (B) Shorten the length of the assessment
    (C) Remove all items that were ambiguous to the clients
    (D) Limit the time the client has to complete the assessment

12. The first kind of prescription medication offered for pain is
    (A) weak opioids
    (B) strong opioids
    (C) NSAIDS (nonsteroidal anti-inflammatory drugs)
    (D) adjuvants

13. The purpose of client assessment is to
    (A) provide feedback on the effectiveness of an intervention program
    (B) place clients in programs based on their needs
    (C) improvement communication between members of the treatment team
    (D) evaluate client performance in therapeutic recreation programs

14. The four basic measurable functions of health (blood pressure, pulse, respiration, and temperature) are called
    (A) vital signs
    (B) health signs
    (C) normal health signs
    (D) normal functioning

15. The CTRS is most likely to work with which of the following disciplines to provide sensory stimulation to individuals with dementia?
    (A) Physical therapy
    (B) Occupational therapy
    (C) Nursing
    (D) Child life

16. When a client has broken her clavicle, she has a broken
    (A) collarbone
    (B) neck
    (C) hip
    (D) leg

17. The purpose of client assessment in therapeutic recreation is to
    (A) identify a client's leisure interests
    (B) make appropriate referrals to various professionals
    (C) gather information to develop an individual treatment plan
    (D) list the client's strengths and weaknesses

18. Which of the following is most likely to produce error in a client's assessment score?
    (A) Lack of confidence in the CTRS
    (B) Inconsistent administration of the assessment tool
    (C) Computerizing the assessment process
    (D) Following an assessment protocol

19. Which of the following are typical parts of a diagnostic protocol?
(A) Assessment, planning, implementation, evaluation
(B) Subjective, objective, analysis, planning
(C) Comprehensive program descriptions and specific program descriptions
(D) Client problems, assessment criteria, process criteria, and outcomes criteria

20. The CTRS runs a community-based disability management program for individuals diagnosed with diabetes. Which of the following is NOT a programming consideration for these individuals?
(A) Monitor blood glucose before and after exercise
(B) Teach participants about diet and nutrition
(C) Teach participants about stress management
(D) Use large print materials with high contrast lettering

21. Alcohol is classified in which of the following categories of drugs?
(A) Stimulants
(B) Depressants
(C) Hallucinogens
(D) Narcotics

22. An older person who does not have static or dynamic balance is at greater risk for
(A) falls
(B) loss of muscle strength
(C) loss of flexibility
(D) loss of endurance

23. Using a strengths-based approach to therapeutic recreation programming means the CTRS
(A) focuses on the abilities of the clients
(B) measures precisely the clients' functional deficits
(C) provides upper-body strengthening and conditioning programs
(D) focuses on the clients' former leisure lifestyles

24. The statement that identifies the agency's basic values and beliefs, and thus defines how it wants to be perceived by the public is called a
(A) mission statement
(B) scope of care statement
(C) marketing statement
(D) external monitoring statement

25. For each of the standards in the *ATRA Standards of Practice*, what elements are included as measurement criteria?
(A) Structure, process, and outcomes
(B) Assessment, planning, implementation, and evaluation
(C) Rating scales from 1 (Very Poor) to 10 (Excellent)
(D) Self-reporting and peer review

26. Therapeutic recreation programs for individuals with acute schizophrenic disorders are MOST appropriate when they focus on goals to improve or increase
(A) social interaction and motor behaviors
(B) integration into community recreation activities
(C) adaptive responses to addictive behaviors
(D) manipulative behaviors of the client

27. Unlike a municipal hospital, a private, for-profit hospital usually
(A) specializes in one or a limited number of disorders
(B) is operated by a governmental entity, such as a county
(C) serves only children
(D) serves individuals on a long-term basis

28. The four axes of the *Diagnostic and Statistical Manual IV-TR* are
(A) physical, social, emotional, and intellectual disorders
(B) clinical disorders, medical disorders, personality disorders, and psychosocial problems
(C) anxiety disorders, affective disorders, substance abuse, and psychomotor disorders
(D) schizophrenia, bi-polar disorder, substance abuse, and depression

29. The national voluntary professional registration program that preceded the National Council for Therapeutic Recreation Certification was administered by the:
(A) National Therapeutic Recreation Society (NTRS)
(B) American Therapeutic Recreation Society (ATRA)
(C) American Association of Recreational Therapy (AART)
(D) Council for the Advancement of Hospital Recreation (CAHR)

30. Medicare Part B provides for all of the following health services EXCEPT
(A) prescription medications
(B) doctors' office visits
(C) out-patient rehabilitation services
(D) medically necessary physical and occupational therapy

31. The primary purpose of a therapeutic recreation service model is to
(A) provide data for comprehensive program development
(B) serve as a guide for the development of programs offered to clients
(C) provide a standard by which programs can be evaluated
(D) distinguish between services provided within various settings

32. The director of the TR department conducted a study on the effectiveness of the previous marketing efforts done for therapeutic recreation services. The action taken by the director is called a marketing _____.
(A) audit
(B) research schema
(C) audience
(D) tool

33. What is the purpose of the Health Protection/Health Promotion Model?
(A) Independent leisure functioning
(B) Facilitating healthy self-actualization
(C) Attaining highest level of health
(D) Reducing blocks to quality of life behaviors

34. Which of the following is NOT a result of chronic stress?
(A) Adrenal glands secrete corticoids that inhibit digestion
(B) Cellular tissue repair is made more quickly
(C) Reproduction system is impaired
(D) Immune system is weakened

35. In the Leisure Ability Model, which of the following would be considered an appropriate goal for functional intervention?
(A) To improve time-on-task
(B) To learn about inexpensive leisure resources in the community
(C) To improve group-entry skills
(D) To participate in a fitness activity of her choice

36. A person who has a(n) _____ disorder may have limited, inflexible behaviors that inhibit his/her ability to interact with others and deal with certain aspects of his/her environment.
(A) circulatory
(B) attention deficit
(C) nervous
(D) orthopedic

37. Patients have the right to have the treatment plan explained to them. According to the *ATRA Code of Ethics*, this principle is called?
(A) Confidentiality and privacy
(B) Justice
(C) Veracity
(D) Informed consent

38. Quality assurance/continuous quality improvement is
(A) a method of comprehensive program evaluation for future program enhancement
(B) a method for implementing in-service staff training
(C) required in all clinical and community agencies
(D) the first step in designing a comprehensive program

39. Using an ecological perspective for therapeutic recreation programming means the CTRS
(A) focuses on the interactions between clients and their environments
(B) teaches clients to reduce, reuse, and recycle
(C) reuses supplies as much as possible
(D) coordinates services with other members of the transdisciplinary team

40. A treatment plan should be entered into the medical chart after
(A) seeing the patient once
(B) conferring with the physician
(C) the patient/legal guardian has agreed to the treatment plan
(D) the patient has been in the hospital for a week

41. One example of a mood disorder is the diagnosis of
(A) psychosis
(B) bipolar personality
(C) paranoia
(D) organic brain syndrome

42. In implementing a leisure education program for four year old children, the CTRS becomes aware that the planned activity requires abstract thought, which the clients are not capable of. The CTRS inadequately analyzed the _____ requirements of the activity for the given population.
(A) social
(B) emotional
(C) physical
(D) cognitive

43. Which social interaction pattern is displayed in singles tennis?
(A) Intragroup
(B) Multilateral
(C) Interindividual
(D) Extraindividual

44. For individuals with disabilities from preschool to the age of 21, a transition plan for services must be in place while they are in school, as required by what piece of federal legislation?
(A) Rehabilitation Act of 1978
(B) Americans with Disabilities Act of 1990
(C) New Freedom Initiative of 2000
(D) Individuals with Disabilities Education Act of 2004

45. The medical term "oriented x3" is the abbreviation for
(A) can go as high as 3 times tables in math skills
(B) recognizes 3 objects
(C) oriented to person, place and time
(D) can have three visitors at a time

46. Which part of the SOAP progress note is the following statement?
"Patient states: "Don't bother me?""
(A) S – Subjective
(B) O – Objective
(C) A – Assessment
(D) P – Plan

47. Networking is helpful to therapeutic recreation specialists because
(A) expertise and ideas are shared to improve the quality of programs
(B) each professional can claim a unique set of skills
(C) clients are not likely to know more than one therapeutic recreation specialist
(D) individuals with disabilities are likely to receive fewer services in the future

48. In which of the four domains does the following statement fall under?
"To ask for assistance when needed"
(A) Cognitive
(B) Affective
(C) Physical
(D) Social

49. In which of the four domains does the following statement fall under?
"To improve ability to locate leisure resources"
(A) Cognitive
(B) Affective
(C) Physical
(D) Social

50. Which statement describes the purpose of evidence-based practice?
(A) Method of designing critical pathways
(B) Process to control medical bills through reduction of services
(C) Means of conducting near-patient research
(D) Method to enhance client care through application of research results

51. The Americans with Disabilities Act includes provisions specifically regarding
(A) employment, government services, and recreation
(B) public transit, government services, and recreation
(C) employment, public entities, telecommunications, and public accommodations
(D) employment, recreation, and public accommodations

52. The CTRS says to the client, "Let's stay in the present and take responsibility for your actions." This specialist is using which type of "therapy" approach?
(A) Gestalt therapy
(B) Rational-emotive therapy
(C) Cognitive therapy
(D) Reality therapy

53. According to *Healthy People 2020*, individuals with disabilities are much more likely to experience all of the following EXCEPT
(A) reduced use of tobacco
(B) increased incidence of obesity
(C) fewer diagnostic and preventative tests
(D) high blood pressure

54. The CTRS asked clients who had recently experienced strokes to identify their highest priorities, set goals, and develop an action plan for their leisure. The technique is called
(A) goal orientation
(B) self-actualization
(C) time management
(D) remotivation

55. High-quality documentation is important for all of the following reasons EXCEPT to
(A) show the patient's leisure history
(B) provide data for quality improvement
(C) improve communication among staff members
(D) provide professional accountability for services rendered

56. Which of the following is a likely result of a profession having and adhering to protocols?
(A) More people are likely to enter the field
(B) The specialist can provide better services that are more similar to others provided around the country
(C) Clients will need to stay in treatment facilities longer to receive the full benefits of the protocol
(D) Insurance companies are likely to deny payment for services in the protocol

57. Observation of overt behavior and the learning of new behavior is a focus of _____ theory.
(A) psychoanalytic
(B) cognitive-behavioral
(C) behavioristic
(D) growth

58. All programs in therapeutic recreation should be based on
(A) resources
(B) client need
(C) client interests
(D) clinician skill

59. The CTRS in a long-term care facility plans on designing a program that maximizes interaction between residents. Which of the following would be a PRIMARY consideration in developing and modifying this program?
(A) Existing social skills of the residents
(B) Available facilities
(C) Necessary equipment and materials
(D) Number of qualified staff

60. The CTRS bases her intervention programs on the notion that all clients desire to interact effectively with their physical and social environments and to view themselves as skilled in their quest for a happy and fulfilling life. She is basing her intervention programs on the theory of
(A) competence-effectance motivation
(B) trust-building
(C) flow
(D) social psychology of leisure

61. Given the goal statement below, which of the following is the most appropriate therapeutic recreation program?
"Goal: To increase clients' independent community skills"
(A) Vacation planning seminar
(B) Instructions on taking the bus
(C) Problem solving discussion group
(D) Social skills functional intervention program

62. Which part of the SOAP note focuses on the CTRS's interpretation of the client's actions and verbalizations?
(A) S – Subjective data
(B) O – Objective data
(C) A – Analysis
(D) P – Plan

63. Which of the following is an appropriate way to resolve conflicts in communication and achieve compromise?
(A) Being aggressive in order to manipulate or intimidate
(B) Negotiating and coming to an agreement
(C) Giving in to avoid unpleasantness
(D) Avoiding the unpleasant person or situation

64. In the classical pattern of multiple sclerosis, the person experiences alternating intervals of
(A) episodes of symptoms and remission
(B) short mania and longer term depression
(C) athetosis and ataxia
(D) muscle atrophy and hypertonia

65. The CTRS was interacting with the client and said," You said you wanted to become more physically active but you refused to come to exercise class today." The CTRS was using which of the following communication techniques?
A) Teach back
(B) Summarization of feeling
(C) Confrontation
(D) Request for clarification

66. Inclusive recreation means that individuals with disabilities
    (A) attend segregated services before attending other programs
    (B) are mixed with individuals with dissimilar disabilities
    (C) are denied access to community programs because special programs are created
    (D) attend recreation programs of choice and have equal and joint participation

67. The CTRS evaluated the 16-week summer programming sessions at 4-week, 8-week, and 12-week intervals to gather which of the following types of program evaluation information?
    (A) Instantaneous time sampling
    (B) Quality assurance health care monitoring
    (C) Formative
    (D) Summative

68. One reason that client assessment is important to therapeutic recreation service delivery is it
    (A) empowers clients to prepare for life changes
    (B) relates directly to program evaluation
    (C) helps clients achieve their goals by being placed in the most appropriate programs
    (D) analyzes which programs are best for certain groups of clients

69. The definition of intellectual disability adopted by the American Association on Intellectual and Developmental Disability (AAIDD) suggests that there is a relationship between intellectual functioning and which of the following?
    (A) Social skills
    (B) Physical skills
    (C) Lability
    (D) Adaptive behavior

70. All of the following are ways to establish rapport with clients in an assessment interview, EXCEPT
    (A) introduce yourself and explain your department
    (B) provide answers for the client
    (C) refer to the client by name
    (D) use body language that signals you are listening

71. One reason that individuals older than 65 experience increased pain is that they
    (A) have more body parts failing
    (B) are unable to report it adequately
    (C) are often unable to speak or gesture
    (D) experience more side effects from numerous prescribed medications

72. The client was discharged from the clinical facility because it was determined that he was not making further progress in his rehabilitation efforts and the "bed space" could be better utilized for an incoming patient. Which of the following committees or departments would make this recommendation?
    (A) Professional standards review organization (PSRO)
    (B) Utilization review
    (C) Medical records review
    (D) Risk management review

73. There are how many vertebrae in the thoracic vertebrae of the human spine?
    (A) 8
    (B) 10
    (C) 12
    (D) 14

74. Which of the following is NOT part of the NCTRC fieldwork requirements (academic path)?
    (A) The on-site fieldwork supervisor must be a CTRS at the beginning of the internship
    (B) The university supervisor must be a CTRS
    (C) A 14-week fieldwork requirement must be completed
    (D) The fieldwork placement must be completed at two different agencies (clinical and community)

75. Those groups of clients known to not benefit from participation will be identified in which part of a protocol?
    (A) Etiology
    (B) Diagnostic criteria
    (C) Inclusion criteria
    (D) Risk management considerations

76. A CTRS should observe all of the following procedures when transferring an individual with a physical disability EXCEPT
    (A) standing with feet together
    (B) asking how and what type of assistance is needed
    (C) maintaining a firm grasp on the individual throughout all points of the transfer
    (D) keeping the majority of the individual's weight as close as possible to the CTRS's own body

77. An assessment protocol increases the likelihood that the assessment will
    (A) be administered the same way every time it is given
    (B) psychometrically sound
    (C) focus on more than leisure and activity interests
    (D) be reliable for a wide variety of clients

78. The CTRS is a supervisor of a large therapeutic recreation department in a community mental health center. When staff cutbacks were ordered in the TR department by the center's administrators, she ignored the memos and continued to staff the units on regular schedules. The conflict resolution strategy employed by The CTRS is called _____.
    (A) avoidance
    (B) defusion
    (C) containment
    (D) confrontation

79. The first step in the assessment implementation process is for the CTRS to
    (A) interpret results for client placement into programs
    (B) analyze or score the assessment results
    (C) administer the assessment to the client
    (D) review the assessment protocol

80. The basic premise behind "managed care" in the health care industry is
    (A) positive client outcomes produced at low cost
    (B) less focus on the individual, more focus on the diagnosis
    (C) sustaining a person's life at all costs
    (D) that insurance companies will pay whatever the clinical facility charges for a service

81. The Leisure Competence Measure (LCM) parallels the format of which of the following client assessments?
    (A) Functional Independence Measure (FIM)
    (B) Rancho Los Amigos Scale
    (C) Brief Leisure Rating Scale (BLRS)
    (D) Leisure Barriers Inventory (LBI)

82. The drug Librium is most often used to treat which of the following disorders?
    (A) Chronic angina
    (B) Anxiety
    (C) Muscle stiffness
    (D) Arrhythmias

83. Which of the following assessments was designed to coincide with the Functional Independence Measure (FIM)?
    (A) Leisure Diagnostic Battery (LDB)
    (B) Comprehensive Evaluation in Recreational Therapy Scale (CERT) – Psych
    (C) Leisure Competence Measure (LCM)
    (D) Leisure Activities Blank (LAB)

84. Evidence-based practice means that the
    (A) CTRS selects interventions based on research findings and professional expertise
    (B) client needs to see evidence before participating
    (C) client is at the center of the treatment
    (D) client will be involved in inclusionary programs

85. An individual's responses or scores on the MDS 3.0 may link to a "trigger" that requires a Care Area Trigger (CAT) to be completed. This means that
    (A) an individual will receive a more in-depth assessment in this area
    (B) the CTRS must complete an interview with the family
    (C) the assessment was completed incorrectly
    (D) the information from the assessment is neither valid or reliable

86. The CTRS wants to teach clients new leisure activities they can do for low- to no-cost in their home. The best group format would be
    (A) Instructional class
    (B) Clubs and special interest groups
    (C) Drop-in center
    (D) Out-trips

87. The CTRS is asked to submit an annual budget that assumes she starts with no dollars and asks her to justify each dollar she then requests. This type of budgeting is called
    (A) zero-based budgeting
    (B) zero-sum score budgeting
    (C) revenue and expense budgeting
    (D) NIL (No Income or Losses) budgeting

88. Diabetic retinopathy is a condition that often results in
    (A) amputation of lower limbs
    (B) higher blood sugar levels
    (C) blindness
    (D) dark spots on the field of vision

89. The results from any assessment should give the CTRS a clear indication of
    (A) the programs in which the client should be placed
    (B) the client's leisure interests
    (C) the validity of the tool
    (D) how successful the client has been in achieving the program outcomes

90. Which statement correctly identifies the criteria of an accessible parking space?
    (A) Accessible parking spaces are closest to the building entrance
    (B) Accessible parking may be distributed in a parking lot if greater access is achieved
    (C) Parking spaces and aisles are level with a slope no greater than 1:20
    (D) Parking spaces are at least 96 inches wide with adjacent access aisle of 68 inches

Practice Test 4

Scoring Sheet

1. Ⓐ Ⓑ Ⓒ Ⓓ   14. Ⓐ Ⓑ Ⓒ Ⓓ   27. Ⓐ Ⓑ Ⓒ Ⓓ   40. Ⓐ Ⓑ Ⓒ Ⓓ

2. Ⓐ Ⓑ Ⓒ Ⓓ   15. Ⓐ Ⓑ Ⓒ Ⓓ   28. Ⓐ Ⓑ Ⓒ Ⓓ   41. Ⓐ Ⓑ Ⓒ Ⓓ

3. Ⓐ Ⓑ Ⓒ Ⓓ   16. Ⓐ Ⓑ Ⓒ Ⓓ   29. Ⓐ Ⓑ Ⓒ Ⓓ   42. Ⓐ Ⓑ Ⓒ Ⓓ

4. Ⓐ Ⓑ Ⓒ Ⓓ   17. Ⓐ Ⓑ Ⓒ Ⓓ   30. Ⓐ Ⓑ Ⓒ Ⓓ   43. Ⓐ Ⓑ Ⓒ Ⓓ

5. Ⓐ Ⓑ Ⓒ Ⓓ   18. Ⓐ Ⓑ Ⓒ Ⓓ   31. Ⓐ Ⓑ Ⓒ Ⓓ   44. Ⓐ Ⓑ Ⓒ Ⓓ

6. Ⓐ Ⓑ Ⓒ Ⓓ   19. Ⓐ Ⓑ Ⓒ Ⓓ   32. Ⓐ Ⓑ Ⓒ Ⓓ   45. Ⓐ Ⓑ Ⓒ Ⓓ

7. Ⓐ Ⓑ Ⓒ Ⓓ   20. Ⓐ Ⓑ Ⓒ Ⓓ   33. Ⓐ Ⓑ Ⓒ Ⓓ   46. Ⓐ Ⓑ Ⓒ Ⓓ

8. Ⓐ Ⓑ Ⓒ Ⓓ   21. Ⓐ Ⓑ Ⓒ Ⓓ   34. Ⓐ Ⓑ Ⓒ Ⓓ   47. Ⓐ Ⓑ Ⓒ Ⓓ

9. Ⓐ Ⓑ Ⓒ Ⓓ   22. Ⓐ Ⓑ Ⓒ Ⓓ   35. Ⓐ Ⓑ Ⓒ Ⓓ   48. Ⓐ Ⓑ Ⓒ Ⓓ

10. Ⓐ Ⓑ Ⓒ Ⓓ   23. Ⓐ Ⓑ Ⓒ Ⓓ   36. Ⓐ Ⓑ Ⓒ Ⓓ   49. Ⓐ Ⓑ Ⓒ Ⓓ

11. Ⓐ Ⓑ Ⓒ Ⓓ   24. Ⓐ Ⓑ Ⓒ Ⓓ   37. Ⓐ Ⓑ Ⓒ Ⓓ   50. Ⓐ Ⓑ Ⓒ Ⓓ

12. Ⓐ Ⓑ Ⓒ Ⓓ   25. Ⓐ Ⓑ Ⓒ Ⓓ   38. Ⓐ Ⓑ Ⓒ Ⓓ   51. Ⓐ Ⓑ Ⓒ Ⓓ

13. Ⓐ Ⓑ Ⓒ Ⓓ   26. Ⓐ Ⓑ Ⓒ Ⓓ   39. Ⓐ Ⓑ Ⓒ Ⓓ   52. Ⓐ Ⓑ Ⓒ Ⓓ

53. Ⓐ Ⓑ Ⓒ Ⓓ   66. Ⓐ Ⓑ Ⓒ Ⓓ   79. Ⓐ Ⓑ Ⓒ Ⓓ

54. Ⓐ Ⓑ Ⓒ Ⓓ   67. Ⓐ Ⓑ Ⓒ Ⓓ   80. Ⓐ Ⓑ Ⓒ Ⓓ

55. Ⓐ Ⓑ Ⓒ Ⓓ   68. Ⓐ Ⓑ Ⓒ Ⓓ   81. Ⓐ Ⓑ Ⓒ Ⓓ

56. Ⓐ Ⓑ Ⓒ Ⓓ   69. Ⓐ Ⓑ Ⓒ Ⓓ   82. Ⓐ Ⓑ Ⓒ Ⓓ

57. Ⓐ Ⓑ Ⓒ Ⓓ   70. Ⓐ Ⓑ Ⓒ Ⓓ   83. Ⓐ Ⓑ Ⓒ Ⓓ

58. Ⓐ Ⓑ Ⓒ Ⓓ   71. Ⓐ Ⓑ Ⓒ Ⓓ   84. Ⓐ Ⓑ Ⓒ Ⓓ

59. Ⓐ Ⓑ Ⓒ Ⓓ   72. Ⓐ Ⓑ Ⓒ Ⓓ   85. Ⓐ Ⓑ Ⓒ Ⓓ

60. Ⓐ Ⓑ Ⓒ Ⓓ   73. Ⓐ Ⓑ Ⓒ Ⓓ   86. Ⓐ Ⓑ Ⓒ Ⓓ

61. Ⓐ Ⓑ Ⓒ Ⓓ   74. Ⓐ Ⓑ Ⓒ Ⓓ   87. Ⓐ Ⓑ Ⓒ Ⓓ

62. Ⓐ Ⓑ Ⓒ Ⓓ   75. Ⓐ Ⓑ Ⓒ Ⓓ   88. Ⓐ Ⓑ Ⓒ Ⓓ

63. Ⓐ Ⓑ Ⓒ Ⓓ   76. Ⓐ Ⓑ Ⓒ Ⓓ   89. Ⓐ Ⓑ Ⓒ Ⓓ

64. Ⓐ Ⓑ Ⓒ Ⓓ   77. Ⓐ Ⓑ Ⓒ Ⓓ   90. Ⓐ Ⓑ Ⓒ Ⓓ

65. Ⓐ Ⓑ Ⓒ Ⓓ   78. Ⓐ Ⓑ Ⓒ Ⓓ

Practice Test 4

Scoring Key

Foundational Knowledge

1. A	16. A	30. A	51. C	66. D	82. B
8. C	20. D	34. B	53. A	69. D	84. A
10. C	21. B	36. B	57. C	71. B	86. A
12. C	26. A	41. B	60. A	73. C	88. C
14. A	28. B	44. D	64. A	76. A	90. B

Practice of TR/RT

2. A	18. B	35. A	46. A	58. B	75. B
4. C	22. A	37. D	48. D	59. A	77. A
5. D	23. A	39. A	49. A	61. B	79. D
7. D	25. A	40. C	50. D	63. B	81. A
11. C	27. A	42. D	52. D	65. C	83. C
13. B	31. B	43. C	54. C	68. C	85. A
17. C	33. C	45. C	56. B	70. B	89. A

Organization of TR/RT

6. D	15. B	24. A	62. C	72. B	80. A
9. C	19. D	55. A	67. C	78. A	87. A

Advancement of the Profession

3. A	29. A	32. A	38. A	47. A	74. D

PRACTICE TEST 4

Record Your Scores Here

Foundational Knowldge   _____ / 30 = _____ %
Practice of TR/RT   _____ / 42 = _____ %
Organization of TR/RT   _____ / 12 = _____ %
Advancement of the Profession _____ / 6 = _____ %

Total Score =   _____ /90
Total Percent = _____ %

If you need more practice in any area(s), proceed to the next practice test.

chapter 10

Practice Test 5

This practice test represents the kind of items you will find on the NCTRC Certification Exam. The purpose of the practice test is to give you some indication of what it will feel like to take the actual NCTRC exam. The length of the test, and the content and format of the questions is close to that of the national test. The 90 items are also in the same proportion as the actual exam, in each of the categories of the Exam Content Outline. See Chapters 2 and 4 for more details about the proportion of items across the four categories of the Exam Content Outline. Additional practice tests follow.

Directions: For each question in this section, select the best of the answer choices given. Use the answer sheet on page 136-137 to record your answers. Use the scoring key on page 138 to score your answers. If you complete the additional practice tests, compare your percentages of correct items in each of the four categories of content. This will give you some idea on which areas you are scoring better and which areas need more work.

1. Which of the following is NOT a principle of activity analysis?
    (A) Analyze the activity as it is normally engaged in
    (B) Analyze the activity with regard to the minimal level of skills required for basic, successful participation
    (C) Complete the activity analysis at least 24 hours before leading the activity
    (D) When completing an activity analysis, rate the activity as compared to all other activities

2. Which one of the four categories of child development does the skill "walks with help" belong?
    (A) Personal/social
    (B) Adaptive/fine motor behavior
    (C) Motor behavior
    (D) Language

3. The CTRS in a facility for at-risk youth plans on designing an anger management skills program. Which of the following would be a PRIMARY consideration in developing and modifying this program?
    (A) Available facilities
    (B) Necessary equipment and materials
    (C) Existing emotional control of the youth
    (D) Existing physical abilities of the youth

4. A person-centered approach to therapeutic recreation means that
    (A) despite differences, we accept that each individual is a unique person
    (B) we encourage age-appropriate behaviors and activities
    (C) we can reduce the impact of the self-fulfilling prophecy
    (D) we encourage clients to think of themselves first, others second

5. Which of the following is the BEST example of public advocacy?
   (A) Speaking on behalf of a patient during a treatment team meeting
   (B) Going to a city council meeting to support additional community access
   (C) Talking with a patient's family about rights and responsibilities
   (D) Making a bulletin board of patients' artwork

6. Down Syndrome, the best-known form of chromosomal intellectual disability, is characterized by
   (A) short stature and enlarged rib cage and upper arms
   (B) flat, broad face and small ears and nose
   (C) increased urinary tract infections and sexual dysfunction
   (D) lowered IQ and osteoporosis

7. In the Leisure Ability Model, which of the following would be considered an appropriate goal under leisure awareness?
   (A) To improve taking personal responsibility for leisure
   (B) To improve cooperative leisure skills
   (C) To actively participate in a conversation for 5 minutes
   (D) To learn about activity opportunities

8. The three major characteristics of intellectual disability are
   (A) subaverage intellectual functioning, impairment in at least two adaptive skill areas, and evident before age 18
   (B) subaverage intellectual functioning, lack of physical coordination skills, and extraordinary facial features
   (C) subaverage social, intellectual, and physical functioning within community expectations
   (D) subaverage functioning in home, community, and school environments

9. Which of the following best represents the Activity Therapy model of therapeutic recreation service delivery?
   (A) The focus of programs is on activity skills acquisition
   (B) Similar disciplines, such as art, music, dance and recreation therapy, are housed in one department
   (C) The philosophy is "All recreation is therapeutic"
   (D) The focus of programs is on improving the functional independence of clients

10. Which of the following conditions is genetic, produces gradually wasting muscle, with accompanying weakness and deformity?
    (A) Spina bifida
    (B) Multiple sclerosis
    (C) Muscular dystrophy
    (D) Osteoarthritis

11. The Centers for Medicare and Medicaid Services requires that the MDS 3.0 assessment be conducted with
    (A) all individuals in mental health facilities
    (B) all individuals in long-term care facilities
    (C) qualified individuals in physical medicine facilities
    (D) individuals over the age of 65 with a confirmed medical disability

12. Active treatment means that intervention is
    (A) delivered in the least restrictive environment
    (B) provided to all clients, regardless of ability and/or interest
    (C) based on reasonable expectation of improving the client's condition and reducing future care
    (D) based on the American College of Sports Medicine's (ACSM's) recommendation for physically active leisure

13. One of the primary precautions for programming for individuals with hearing impairments is a secondary condition of
    (A) balance deficits
    (B) lowered intelligence
    (C) obesity
    (D) astigmatism

14. All of the following are examples of leisure barriers measured in the Leisure Barrier Inventory, EXCEPT
    (A) time, money, and transportation
    (B) poor self-concept
    (C) availability of leisure partners
    (D) understanding of leisure as a concept

15. A client was rated by his physician as having a 61-70 score on the Global Assessment of Functioning (GAF). The CTRS knew that this might mean the client would benefit from the following services?
    (A) Activities of daily living and community Integration
    (B) Decision-making, problem solving, and coping skills
    (C) Functional improvement, time management, and stress management
    (D) Health prevention and stress coping

16. Mental illness may be considered any disorder that
   (A) is congenital and transient
   (B) results from lower intellectual capacity and lower adaptive behavior
   (C) results in abnormal behavior that can be seen as bizarre, unusual, and irritating
   (D) exhibits alteration of thought, mood or behavior so that the individual has difficulty meeting daily living requirements

17. Listed below are four steps to "thought stopping."
   1. Imagine the thought
   2. Unaided thought interruption
   3. Aided thought interruption
   4. Thought substitution

   Which of the following correctly orders these steps from first to last?
   (A) 1, 2, 3, 4
   (B) 1, 3, 2, 4
   (C) 4, 3, 1, 2
   (D) 4, 3, 2, 1

18. Of the five major life areas (vocational, family, spiritual, social, leisure, and legal), leisure often is the _____ impacted by the use of substances.
   (A) last
   (B) second
   (C) first
   (D) third

19. In a facility that adopts the Health Protection/ Health Promotion model, what is the primary purpose of the intervention?
   (A) To provide therapist-directed experiences with clients
   (B) To motivate clients to function independently in the community
   (C) To promote behaviors that enable clients to move toward mastery of their own health
   (D) To enhance leisure decision-making so clients develop self and leisure awareness

20. Typical experiences of individuals with new spinal cord injuries include
   (A) heightened ability to cope with stress, fewer leisure options, and lowered self-esteem
   (B) decreased helplessness, fewer employment opportunities, and better relationships
   (C) loss of ability and skills, disruption of relationships, and dependence on others
   (D) higher risk for infections, lowered intellectual ability, and lowered self-esteem

21. Asking the question, "How stable is the instrument over a given period of time?" is an example of looking at the assessment's
   (A) concurrent validity statistics
   (B) test-retest estimates
   (C) Cronbach's alpha
   (D) internal consistency estimates

22. The federal law (and later amendments) that dictates currently the specifications for barrier free design is the
   (A) Architectural Barriers Act of 1968
   (B) Americans With Disabilities Act of 1990
   (C) Mandatory Inclusion Act of 1992
   (D) Barrier Free Environments Act of 2012

23. Which organization oversees the accreditation of physical medicine programs?
   (A) Joint Commission (JCAHO)
   (B) Rehabilitation Accreditation Commission (CARF)
   (C) American Therapeutic Recreation Association (ATRA)
   (D) Centers for Medicare and Medicaid Services (CMS)

24. When a client has a "lack of leisure awareness," it means she
   (A) knows very few leisure skills
   (B) has severe cognitive deficits
   (C) does not understand the importance of leisure
   (D) has developed a meaningful and satisfying leisure lifestyle

25. During client assessments, the CTRS makes sure to respect the client's viewpoint, allows the client to finish her/his thoughts before speaking again, and asks for clarification when she does not understand an answer. The CTRS is using the technique known as
   (A) values clarification
   (B) active listening
   (C) cognitive restructuring
   (D) non-violent communication

26. Substance addictions are likely to affect a person's leisure lifestyle in which of the following ways?
   (A) Improved social relationships with friends and family
   (B) Reduced need for coping and anger management skills
   (C) Improved energy and intrinsically motivated leisure involvement
   (D) Reduced enjoyment from non-addiction activities

27. The "day-to-day behavioral expression of one's leisure-related attitudes, awareness, and activities revealed within the context and composite of the total life experience" is a person's
(A) leisure lifestyle
(B) recreation well being
(C) quality of life
(D) leisure well being

28. Which of the following activities has been proven to be most effective with improving psychological states?
(A) Soothing music
(B) Building bird houses
(C) Physical exercise
(D) Joining a social club

29. Which of the following should the CTRS do before she interviews the client for the therapeutic recreation assessment?
(A) Decide which behaviors are pertinent to the therapeutic recreation assessment
(B) Perform an activity analysis on likely activities of interest
(C) Review medical records to obtain background information
(D) Interview the clients' family members

30. One leadership principle the CTRS should follow when working with autistic children is to
(A) establish eye contact
(B) use lengthy activities
(C) play a lot of active games
(D) change activities quickly

31. All of the following are true statements about client assessment in therapeutic recreation EXCEPT assessments should be
(A) selected or developed based on a specific purpose
(B) able to gather necessary information in a logical and straightforward manner
(C) able to be completed by clients within a short time frame
(D) able to produce results that are as valid and reliable as possible

32. One of the major DISADVANTAGES of using interviews in client assessment is
(A) unless the scoring system is in place ahead of time, they are difficult to score and analyze
(B) they are less likely to get correct information than observations
(C) that clients often lie about their leisure participation patterns prior to admission
(D) they reduce personal contact between the client and the CTRS

33. When an individual has mild to strong cravings for a substance and believes the substance is necessary to maintain an optimal state of well-being, it is called
(A) drug abuse
(B) psychological dependence
(C) physical dependence
(D) tolerance

34. The Fox Activity Therapy Social Skills Baseline assessment was developed for use with which population?
(A) Older individuals in nursing homes
(B) Adults with developmental disabilities
(C) Adults with mental health disturbances
(D) Disabled children in inclusion programs

35. In the mental illness diagnosis classification system used by the American Psychiatric Association, Axes I and II describe
(A) physical disorders related to mental illness
(B) unrelated symptoms
(C) categories and conditions of mental illness
(D) social support networks that can be used by the client

36. The CTRS wants to assess clients' sensory abilities in functional areas such as visual acuity, depth perception, auditory acuity, and tactile sensation. The best assessment instrument for this use might be the:
(A) Global Assessment of Functioning (GAF)
(B) Comprehensive Evaluation in Recreation Therapy – Physical Disabilities (CERT-PD)
(C) FOX Assessment
(D) Functional Assessment of Therapeutic Recreation Skills

37. In which of the following steps does the CTRS develop intervention protocols?
(A) Assessment
(B) Program planning
(C) Program implementation
(D) Program evaluation

38. The CTRS wants to assess clients' stress management skills. Which of the following questions is most appropriate?
(A) Can you feel the breath going in and out of your body?
(B) When is the last time you experienced stress?
(C) How do you handle stress when you experience it?
(D) Are you aware of stress?

39. Because of efforts to reduce the amount of time individuals spend in in-patient acute care, they are often moved more quickly to
(A) group homes
(B) halfway houses
(C) rehabilitation units or hospitals
(D) health clinics

40. The CTRS wants to assess social skills. Which of the following questions is most appropriate?
(A) What do you like to do when you're alone?
(B) What do you do for fun?
(C) How would you greet someone you do not know?
(D) Do you enjoy dual sports?

41. The CTRS took client medical records home so she could finish her charting for the week. The CTRS is in violation of which law?
(A) Health Insurance Portability and Accountability Act (HIPAA)
(B) American with Disabilities Act
(C) Consumer Health Protection Act
(D) Health Maintenance Organization Act

42. Which of the following is NOT a way for clients to improve their health and well-being?
(A) Exercise to the point of exhaustion once per day
(B) Break patterns of unsatisfying or destructive behaviors
(C) Maximize positive and pleasant experiences
(D) Reflect on positive occurrences in their lives

43. One of the most typical ways to receive direct reimbursement for TR services is by "time units." This means that the patient is charged
(A) per time intervals (e.g., per 15 minutes)
(B) as part of the per diem rate
(C) by the procedures performed
(D) by the hospital's daily bed rate

44. The client has been diagnosed with schizophrenia and admitted as an inpatient. The CTRS should be aware of which of the following possible complications of schizophrenia?
(A) Difficulty participating in groups
(B) Increased resting heart rate
(C) Autonomic dysreflexia
(D) Grand mal seizures

45. The client has been diagnosed with heroin addiction and admitted as an inpatient. The CTRS should be aware of which of the following possible complications of heroin addiction?
(A) Exposure to HIV (human immunodeficiency virus)
(B) Blunted feelings
(C) Rapidly alternating periods of mania and depression
(D) Decreased pain tolerance

46. Continually striving to upgrade one's knowledge and skills necessary to practice proficiently is the definition of
(A) in-service training
(B) continuing professional competence
(C) quality improvement
(D) clinical supervision

47. Which part of the SOAP progress note is the following statement?
"Patient turns away when others try to talk with him/her and attends to a craft or a book."
(A) S – Subjective
(B) O – Objective
(C) A – Assessment
(D) P – Plan

48. Which of the following is NOT a principle of activity selection to address client outcomes?
(A) Activities must have a direct relationship to the client goal
(B) Consider the types of activities in which people will engage when they have choice
(C) Program to the client's outcomes and priorities
(D) Provide large group entertainment activities as often as possible

49. Which of the following are NOT minimal expectations of all therapeutic recreation specialists?
(A) Read professional journals, attend professional conferences, and network
(B) Retain professional certification and join appropriate professional organizations
(C) Study external accreditation documents and professional standards
(D) Maintain professional knowledge as it was at graduation

50. In a leisure skills acquisition class, which of the following activities is usually most appropriate for an adolescent male with a recent thoracic spinal cord injury?
(A) Building remote-controlled model airplanes
(B) Plant care
(C) Pilates
(D) Crossword puzzles

51. Debriefing a therapeutic recreation activity or session is important because it allows clients time to
(A) socialize with peers so the specialist can make additional systematic observations
(B) analyze the intent of the activity and draw conclusions about their own behavior
(C) think about the purpose of the activity and how it relates to their past
(D) take control of the activity and decide what rules and regulations will be followed

52. It is the responsibility of every CTRS to advocate for the leisure rights of individuals with disabilities because leisure is a(n)
(A) privilege
(B) option
(C) right
(D) challenge

53. Which of the following is NOT a characteristic of an outcome-oriented intervention?
(A) All clients receive all services
(B) Systematic design occurs before implementation
(C) Programs area based on individual client need
(D) Outcomes have relevance and importance to the client

54. Which of the following statements indicates that the client is at the precontemplation stage of behavior change?
(A) I'll check out the fitness center when the weather gets nicer.
(B) I'm glad I asked my friend to go to the fitness with me next week.
(C) I don't need to go to a fitness center; I'm in pretty good shape.
(D) I wonder what the hours of the fitness center are?

55. Which of the following is an example of a multi-disciplinary treatment team?
(A) Each team member independently assesses and plans interventions for the client
(B) Each team member is responsible for collaborating with others on identifying common goal areas; then selects the best intervention within his or her discipline
(C) Each team member works across disciplinary boundaries to develop goals and plans, and often co-treats clients
(D) Each team member is cross-trained in each other's discipline and there are virtually no boundaries between disciplines

56. In a leisure resources session, the CTRS, asked the client, "How would you locate a fitness center in your hometown?" The CTRS's question is at what level of Bloom's Cognitive Taxonomy?
(A) Knowledge
(B) Comprehension
(C) Evaluation
(D) Analysis

57. Which of the following is an appropriate strategy for working with individuals with intellectual disabilities?
(A) Present the activity in small steps
(B) Speak loudly and enunciate words clearly
(C) Provide a high degree of stimulation through all five senses
(D) Move through the activity quickly to keep their attention

58.   Which of the following is a TRUE statement about evidence-based practice?
(A) It has been practiced by therapeutic recreation specialists since the early 1990s
(B) It decreases accountability for services provided
(C) The specialist depends on theory-based programming and systems design
(D) Client outcomes are more likely to be achieved when best practices are used

59.   Which of the following client descriptions BEST demonstrates the custodial or long-term care model of service delivery?
(A) Individuals in acute psychiatric care
(B) Day camp participants
(C) Residents in a state mental health facility
(D) Individuals in a physical medicine and rehabilitation center

60.   In a leisure awareness session, the CTRS asked the client, "What skills and abilities contribute to your ability to have fun?" The CTRS's question is at what level of Bloom's Cognitive Taxonomy?
(A) Knowledge
(B) Comprehension
(C) Application
(D) Analysis

61.   In which of the four domains does the following statement fall under? "To improve decision-making skills related to leisure involvement"
(A) Cognitive
(B) Affective
(C) Physical
(D) Social

62.   The largest federal third-party payer in the United States is
(A) Medicare
(B) Blue Cross/Blue Shield
(C) State Farm Insurance
(D) Medicaid

63.   The CTRS used a paper and pencil leisure education activity for a chronic mental health group. During the beginning of the activity, the CTRS realized that the clients could not read. The CTRS did not adequately analyze the _____ requirements of the activity.
(A) cognitive
(B) affective
(C) physical
(D) administrative

64.   The purpose of *Healthy People 2020* is to
(A) establish benchmarks for monitoring the health of U.S. citizens
(B) document an exercise plan that all citizens can easily follow
(C) document nutrition and exercise plan according to individuals' race, age, and gender
(D) provide a cross-country comparison for monitoring the health of the US versus other countries

65.   Problem-oriented medical records have which of the following advantages over source-oriented medical records?
(A) An unrestricted style and format
(B) Improved ability to track problem areas and successes
(C) Record of behavior change over time
(D) Decreases need for staff communication

66.   During a leisure education discussion group, the client sits slumped in his chair with his arms folded and legs crossed. Using non-verbal communication cues, the CTRS assumes that the client is
(A) actively engaged in the activity
(B) becoming overtly aggressive to other patients/clients
(C) disinterested and unengaged in the activity
(D) demonstrating a "closed" position to further communication

67.   The Americans with Disabilities Act requires that public and commercial access be provided in what order of priority?
1   Public sidewalks, parking, or public transportation
2   Areas where goods and services are made available to the public
3   Access to and usability of restroom facilities
4   Any other features necessary to provide access to the goods, services, facilities, privileges, advantages, or accommodations of a place of public accommodation
(A) 1, 2, 3, 4
(B) 3, 2, 1, 4
(C) 4, 3, 2, 1
(D) 3, 1, 2, 4

68. When serving a program evaluation function, the assessment tool or procedure and its results may be used to
(A) plan appropriate programs for client needs
(B) provide an accurate and valid diagnosis for client treatment
(C) monitor the continuing behavior of clients
(D) ask for input from the other therapists on the treatment team

69. According to the Transtheoretical Model, if the client has developed a plan of action with intentions for implementation within the next month, he is at what stage of behavior change?
(A) Precontemplation
(B) Contemplation
(C) Preparation
(D) Action

70. A marketing audit is a vital step in designing a marketing plan for a therapeutic recreation department because it
(A) describes what past marketing efforts and effects have been
(B) evaluates the target audiences and the information they seek
(C) critiques what others have done in the area
(D) establishes goals and objectives for implementation

71. Which of the following examples demonstrates the concept of "flow?"
(A) The client got so involved in painting a sunset, she lost track of time
(B) The client, after trying a number of activities, decides he likes archery the best
(C) The client has three cats and two dogs and volunteers at the animal shelter twice a week
(D) The client likes to travel to new places at least twice a year

72. The major difference between an acute care hospital and a physical rehabilitation center is the
(A) types of professionals found on the treatment team
(B) patient's/client's readiness for outpatient programs
(C) patient's/client's medical stability and need for care
(D) level of professional accountability required by external accreditation standards

73. Which of the following is NOT criteria for selecting "important aspects of care" to monitor during quality assurance reviews?
(A) Programs that serve large numbers of clients
(B) Programs that put clients at risk of serious consequences
(C) Programs that occur on an annual basis
(D) Programs that, in the past, have produced problems for staff or clients

74. A client's symptoms of irritability, pallor, trembling, blurred vision, perspiration, fatigue, confusion and headache, may be indicators of
(A) traumatic brain injury
(B) diabetic coma
(C) heart attack
(D) post-traumatic stress syndrome

75. In medical terminology, AROM means
(A) about the room once
(B) asynchronous range of motion
(C) active range of motion
(D) higher than average

76. Which of the following statements is TRUE about the following objective?
"After completion of the Social Skills Program, the client will introduce herself to one other peer, using the five-step procedure as instructed."
(A) The condition is missing
(B) The behavior is missing
(C) The criterion is missing
(D) The objective is complete as is

77. Which of the following is a TRUE statement regarding pain?
(A) Pain medications cause addictions
(B) Young children do not experience pain
(C) If a child can be distracted, he is not in pain
(D) Slightly less than half of hospitalized children experience pain

78. A written plan of operation for a therapeutic recreation department is most similar to a
(A) policy and procedure manual
(B) description of the department's quality performance 'nitiatives
(C) personnel maintenance record
(D) summary of all departmental risk management activities for the past five years

79. In the Leisure Ability Model, which of the following would be considered an appropriate goal under leisure resources?
    (A) To improve taking personal responsibility for leisure
    (B) To gain an understanding of the effects of disability or illness on leisure behavior
    (C) To provide leisure opportunities that allows the client freedom to voluntarily participate
    (D) To locate a low-cost fitness activity in the community

80. Which of the following is a team-building strategy for personnel within a therapeutic recreation department?
    (A) Establish goals that are to be accomplished as a group
    (B) Implement policies without staff input
    (C) Keep the information flow to a minimum
    (D) Make unilateral decisions

81. A typical secondary condition to osteoarthritis is
    (A) anxiety
    (B) decubitus ulcers
    (C) obesity
    (D) joint pain

82. In health care, the term "capitation" means the health care provider
    (A) agrees to a preset dollar amount per person and to not ask for further reimbursement
    (B) is reimbursed only for expenses that the client can pay for
    (C) must itemize all charges on the bill and relate each to a specific diagnosis code
    (D) is a member of a fee-for-service organization that agrees on charges prior to admission

83. A _____ is a document kept within a client's medical record that specifies the actions to be taken on the behalf of and by the client in order to reach his goals.
    (A) critical pathway
    (B) written plan of operation
    (C) protocol
    (D) treatment plan

84. The medical term "ad. lib." is the abbreviation for
    (A) as patient can tolerate
    (B) give freedom liberally
    (C) as often as possible
    (D) daily

85. Individuals with spina bifida may be susceptible to a secondary condition called
    (A) cleft palate
    (B) decubitus ulcers
    (C) hip fracture
    (D) synovial distension

86. In calculating the price to be charged the client in a fee-for-service arrangement, the CTRS should consider which of the following costs?
    (A) Direct costs, indirect costs, and uncollectibles (individuals unable to pay)
    (B) Department budget, divided by the number of therapeutic recreation programs
    (C) Department budget, divided by the number of therapeutic recreation staff
    (D) Staff salaries, facility rental, overhead costs

87. Interventions targeted for a specific client are described in a
    (A) clinical or critical pathway
    (B) written plan of operation
    (C) treatment protocol
    (D) treatment plan

88. The therapeutic recreation specialist who knows about personal choice, self-efficacy, and personal causation would do the following while facilitating programs for clients?
    (A) Call the community facility to make arrangements and pay for tickets
    (B) Post a calendar with the month's events listed on a weekly basis
    (C) Help participants finish their projects before leaving the activity room
    (D) Ask participants to help plan the next week's activity session

89. Which of the following is an example of "subjective" data that may be recorded in a progress note?
    (A) The client has a prominent odor late in the day
    (B) The client's sister said, "He doesn't really look forward to getting out"
    (C) The client seems really happy during therapeutic recreation activities
    (D) The client appears depressed and withdrawn

90. A "good" progress note allows for
    (A) considerations of physical, social, intellectual, and emotional aspects
    (B) demonstration of a clear relationship between goals, objectives, and plan of action
    (C) an information update from the assessment and treatment plan
    (D) all of the above

Practice Test 5

Scoring Sheet

1. Ⓐ Ⓑ Ⓒ Ⓓ	14. Ⓐ Ⓑ Ⓒ Ⓓ	27. Ⓐ Ⓑ Ⓒ Ⓓ	40. Ⓐ Ⓑ Ⓒ Ⓓ
2. Ⓐ Ⓑ Ⓒ Ⓓ	15. Ⓐ Ⓑ Ⓒ Ⓓ	28. Ⓐ Ⓑ Ⓒ Ⓓ	41. Ⓐ Ⓑ Ⓒ Ⓓ
3. Ⓐ Ⓑ Ⓒ Ⓓ	16. Ⓐ Ⓑ Ⓒ Ⓓ	29. Ⓐ Ⓑ Ⓒ Ⓓ	42. Ⓐ Ⓑ Ⓒ Ⓓ
4. Ⓐ Ⓑ Ⓒ Ⓓ	17. Ⓐ Ⓑ Ⓒ Ⓓ	30. Ⓐ Ⓑ Ⓒ Ⓓ	43. Ⓐ Ⓑ Ⓒ Ⓓ
5. Ⓐ Ⓑ Ⓒ Ⓓ	18. Ⓐ Ⓑ Ⓒ Ⓓ	31. Ⓐ Ⓑ Ⓒ Ⓓ	44. Ⓐ Ⓑ Ⓒ Ⓓ
6. Ⓐ Ⓑ Ⓒ Ⓓ	19. Ⓐ Ⓑ Ⓒ Ⓓ	32. Ⓐ Ⓑ Ⓒ Ⓓ	45. Ⓐ Ⓑ Ⓒ Ⓓ
7. Ⓐ Ⓑ Ⓒ Ⓓ	20. Ⓐ Ⓑ Ⓒ Ⓓ	33. Ⓐ Ⓑ Ⓒ Ⓓ	46. Ⓐ Ⓑ Ⓒ Ⓓ
8. Ⓐ Ⓑ Ⓒ Ⓓ	21. Ⓐ Ⓑ Ⓒ Ⓓ	34. Ⓐ Ⓑ Ⓒ Ⓓ	47. Ⓐ Ⓑ Ⓒ Ⓓ
9. Ⓐ Ⓑ Ⓒ Ⓓ	22. Ⓐ Ⓑ Ⓒ Ⓓ	35. Ⓐ Ⓑ Ⓒ Ⓓ	48. Ⓐ Ⓑ Ⓒ Ⓓ
10. Ⓐ Ⓑ Ⓒ Ⓓ	23. Ⓐ Ⓑ Ⓒ Ⓓ	36. Ⓐ Ⓑ Ⓒ Ⓓ	49. Ⓐ Ⓑ Ⓒ Ⓓ
11. Ⓐ Ⓑ Ⓒ Ⓓ	24. Ⓐ Ⓑ Ⓒ Ⓓ	37. Ⓐ Ⓑ Ⓒ Ⓓ	50. Ⓐ Ⓑ Ⓒ Ⓓ
12. Ⓐ Ⓑ Ⓒ Ⓓ	25. Ⓐ Ⓑ Ⓒ Ⓓ	38. Ⓐ Ⓑ Ⓒ Ⓓ	51. Ⓐ Ⓑ Ⓒ Ⓓ
13. Ⓐ Ⓑ Ⓒ Ⓓ	26. Ⓐ Ⓑ Ⓒ Ⓓ	39. Ⓐ Ⓑ Ⓒ Ⓓ	52. Ⓐ Ⓑ Ⓒ Ⓓ

53. Ⓐ Ⓑ Ⓒ Ⓓ   66. Ⓐ Ⓑ Ⓒ Ⓓ   79. Ⓐ Ⓑ Ⓒ Ⓓ

54. Ⓐ Ⓑ Ⓒ Ⓓ   67. Ⓐ Ⓑ Ⓒ Ⓓ   80. Ⓐ Ⓑ Ⓒ Ⓓ

55. Ⓐ Ⓑ Ⓒ Ⓓ   68. Ⓐ Ⓑ Ⓒ Ⓓ   81. Ⓐ Ⓑ Ⓒ Ⓓ

56. Ⓐ Ⓑ Ⓒ Ⓓ   69. Ⓐ Ⓑ Ⓒ Ⓓ   82. Ⓐ Ⓑ Ⓒ Ⓓ

57. Ⓐ Ⓑ Ⓒ Ⓓ   70. Ⓐ Ⓑ Ⓒ Ⓓ   83. Ⓐ Ⓑ Ⓒ Ⓓ

58. Ⓐ Ⓑ Ⓒ Ⓓ   71. Ⓐ Ⓑ Ⓒ Ⓓ   84. Ⓐ Ⓑ Ⓒ Ⓓ

59. Ⓐ Ⓑ Ⓒ Ⓓ   72. Ⓐ Ⓑ Ⓒ Ⓓ   85. Ⓐ Ⓑ Ⓒ Ⓓ

60. Ⓐ Ⓑ Ⓒ Ⓓ   73. Ⓐ Ⓑ Ⓒ Ⓓ   86. Ⓐ Ⓑ Ⓒ Ⓓ

61. Ⓐ Ⓑ Ⓒ Ⓓ   74. Ⓐ Ⓑ Ⓒ Ⓓ   87. Ⓐ Ⓑ Ⓒ Ⓓ

62. Ⓐ Ⓑ Ⓒ Ⓓ   75. Ⓐ Ⓑ Ⓒ Ⓓ   88. Ⓐ Ⓑ Ⓒ Ⓓ

63. Ⓐ Ⓑ Ⓒ Ⓓ   76. Ⓐ Ⓑ Ⓒ Ⓓ   89. Ⓐ Ⓑ Ⓒ Ⓓ

64. Ⓐ Ⓑ Ⓒ Ⓓ   77. Ⓐ Ⓑ Ⓒ Ⓓ   90. Ⓐ Ⓑ Ⓒ Ⓓ

65. Ⓐ Ⓑ Ⓒ Ⓓ   78. Ⓐ Ⓑ Ⓒ Ⓓ

Practice Test 5

Scoring Key

Foundational Knowledge

2. C	13. A	24. C	35. C	59. C	74. B
4. A	16. D	26. D	52. C	64. A	77. D
6. B	18. C	28. C	53. A	67. A	81. D
8. A	20. C	30. A	54. C	69. C	85. B
10. C	22. B	33. B	57. A	71. A	88. D

Practice of TR/RT

1. C	15. B	31. C	44. A	58. D	76. D
3. C	17. B	32. A	45. A	60. D	79. D
7. A	19. C	34. B	47. B	61. A	83. D
9. B	21. B	36. B	48. D	63. A	84. A
11. B	25. B	38. C	50. A	66. D	87. D
12. C	27. A	40. C	51. B	72. C	89. B
14. B	29. C	42. A	56. B	75. C	90. D

Organization of TR/RT

37. B	43. A	62. A	68. C	78. A	82. A
39. D	55. A	65. B	73. C	80. A	86. A

Advancement of the Profession

5. B	23. B	41. A	46. B	49. D	70. A

PRACTICE TEST 5

Record Your Scores Here

Foundational Knowledge	_____ / 30 =	_____	%
Practice of TR/RT	_____ / 42 =	_____	%
Organization of TR/RT	_____ / 12 =	_____	%
Advancement of the Profession	_____ / 6 =	_____	%

Total Score = _____ /90

Total Percent = _____ %

If you need more practice in any area(s), proceed to the next practice test.

chapter 11

Practice Test 6

This practice test represents the kind of items you will find on the NCTRC Certification Exam. The purpose of the practice test is to give you some indication of what it will feel like to take the actual NCTRC exam. The length of the test, and the content and format of the questions is close to that of the national test. The 90 items are also in the same proportion as the actual exam, in each of the categories of the Exam Content Outline. See Chapter 2 for more details about the proportion of items across the four categories of the Exam Content Outline.

Directions: For each question in this section, select the best of the answer choices given. Use the answer sheet on pages 149-150 to record your answers. Use the scoring key on page 151 to score your answers. If you complete the additional practice tests, compare your percentages of correct items in each of the four categories of content. This will give you some idea on which areas you are scoring better and which areas need more work.

1. In the Therapeutic Recreation Service Delivery Model, as the client gains in ability to make rational choices and become independent, the CTRS
    (A) reduces control over the intervention
    (B) provides a greater number of community integration activities
    (C) focuses to a greater degree on the client's functional abilities
    (D) switches focus to quality of life

2. What is likely to be the nature/role of CTRS in an acute care setting where the medical model is the mode of operation?
    (A) Design recreation participation programs for evening/weekend participation
    (B) Conduct one-on-one sessions with clients using leisure as a diversionary tool
    (C) Prepare individualized treatment programs based on physician's orders
    (D) Plan leisure education sessions so clients gain an awareness of leisure and life satisfaction

3. For which group of clients is recreation participation programs most suited?
    (A) Clients who need to improve physical well-being and health
    (B) Clients who need to develop new leisure time skills
    (C) Clients who need to develop functional skills
    (D) Clients who need to practice interaction skills in supervised situations

4. During a planning session for a community outing, the CTRS told the group that each person was a team member and was responsible for making decisions and helping to plan the outing. The CTRS was using which of the following types of leadership style?
    (A) Autocratic
    (B) Democratic
    (C) Laissez-faire
    (D) Motivational

5. Which of the following is the BEST example of self-advocacy by someone with a mental illness?
   (A) Responding to a newspaper article saying that mental health services are a waste of money with facts about recovery
   (B) Going to the supermarket to buy groceries
   (C) Joining a weekly support group for individuals with mental illness
   (D) Bringing toys to a children's residential facility during the annual Holiday Toy Drive

6. The CTRS can make which of the following assumptions about clients in a day care center for older adults?
   (A) They are in need of acute medical care
   (B) They have or can arrange transportation and have a reasonable level of health
   (C) They live below the income poverty level
   (D) They need reality orientation and remotivation training activities

7. In 2001, the World Health Organization defined quality of life as
   (A) return to health after a lengthy period of illness or disability
   (B) a person's perception of their overall health and well-being
   (C) the achievement of homeostasis
   (D) a major factor in ratings of patient satisfaction with health care services

8. The client, a 13-year-old boy, has been diagnosed with autism. The CTRS should be aware of which of the following possible effects of autism on leisure activity participation?
   (A) Reduced tolerance for heat
   (B) Inability to stay awake during activities
   (C) Strong need for multiple play partners
   (D) Inability to communicate preferences

9. Focus charting is used when the treatment team wants to
   (A) show similarities and differences between clients
   (B) use a critical care map of client progress
   (C) follow the diagnostic protocol
   (D) emphasize an event, behavior, or circumstance in clients' records

10. The Functional Assessment of Characteristics for Therapeutic Recreation – Revised (FACTR-R) makes which of the following assumptions about physical functional abilities such as vision, hearing, ambulation, and bowel/bladder control?
    (A) Individuals with severe impairments in these areas may not be appropriate for therapeutic recreation services.
    (B) Therapeutic recreation specialists should not be measuring these areas.
    (C) Functional abilities are prerequisite to leisure decision-making.
    (D) Some functional abilities are not amenable to improvement, but are important considerations for TR programming.

11. Which of the following would be typical topics for specific program evaluation questions?
    (A) Content of the assessment and content of the program
    (B) Seasonal program offerings and timing of events
    (C) Validity and reliability of the specific program evaluation questions
    (D) Appropriateness of program content and process for clients who participated

12. Which of the following example demonstrates the concept of "learned helplessness?"
    (A) The client plans on her calendar to do at least one fun thing per week
    (B) The client has repeatedly failed and doesn't want to try any more
    (C) The client has trouble remembering to ask for help
    (D) The client learned that asking for help is not a weakness

13. In what document would the CTRS be MOST likely to find information on staff benefits?
    (A) Quality improvement records
    (B) Policy and procedure manual
    (C) Intern manual
    (D) Personnel files

14. One of the principles in *ATRA's Code of Ethics* is Informed Consent. This concept means
    (A) all client data must be verified by a third party prior to any treatment
    (B) insurance companies have the right to limit the amount of payment for any service
    (C) clients have the right to know the benefits and risks prior to participation
    (D) clients' photographs cannot be taken with their permission

15. If a client receives treatment and was not informed of risks involved and the treatment results in some unwanted side effect or injury, then the client can bring a lawsuit against the CTRS. The CTRS could be found
    (A) guilty of negligence
    (B) having a breach of confidentiality
    (C) to be harmful to all
    (D) guilty of malfeasance

16. Substance-related disorders are categorized according to which Axis in the *Diagnostic and Statistical Manual IV-TR*?
    (A) Axis I – Clinical Disorders
    (B) Axis II – Personality Disorders; Mental Retardation
    (C) Axis III – Acute Medical Conditions
    (D) Axis IV – Psychosocial and Environmental Problems

17. The CTRS was interviewing the client and said, "I'm not sure what you mean by that. Can you explain it to me?" The CTRS was using which of the following communication techniques?
    (A) Teach back
    (B) Summarization of feeling
    (C) Confrontation
    (D) Request for clarification

18. Obsessive-compulsive disorder is categorized according to which Axis in the *Diagnostic and Statistical Manual IV-TR*?
    (A) Axis I – Clinical Disorders
    (B) Axis II – Personality Disorders; Mental Retardation
    (C) Axis III – Acute Medical Conditions
    (D) Axis IV – Psychosocial and Environmental Problems

19. During an assessment interview, the client stated, "I hate physical activities. They just wear me out. But my sister just loves to be involved in sports." The CTRS responded, "You don't like exercise, while your sister does." The CTRS was using which of the following communication techniques?
    (A) Probe
    (B) Summarization
    (C) Redirection
    (D) Confrontation

20. Which of the following is an example of an interdisciplinary treatment team?
    (A) Each team member independently assesses and plans interventions for the client
    (B) Each team member is responsible for collaborating with others on identifying common goal areas; then selects the best intervention within his or her discipline
    (C) Each team member works across disciplinary boundaries to develop goals and plans, and often co-treats clients
    (D) Each team member is cross-trained in each other's discipline and there are virtually no boundaries between disciplines

21. The CTRS wants to help clients with mental health issues increase physical flexibility. What activity is most appropriate for this purpose?
    (A) Yoga
    (B) Volleyball
    (C) Softball
    (D) Core training

22. Which of the following activities is most appropriate for improving clients' knowledge of the benefits of leisure?
    (A) Social interaction skill instruction
    (B) Knowledge of leisure resources
    (C) Leisure awareness
    (D) Leisure interest exploration

23. Therapeutic recreation services are often included in a facility's per diem rate which means that services are
    (A) directly billable in 15-minute increments
    (B) part of one daily charge for allowable costs
    (C) established on a case-by-case basis
    (D) discounted for large groups negotiated by the insurance company

24. A CTRS wants to assess a patient's/client's ability to follow simple directions. The CTRS should assess behavior from which of the following domains?
    (A) Cognitive
    (B) Physical
    (C) Emotional
    (D) Social

25. Which of the following is NOT a primary symptom of substance use disorders?
   (A) Inability to distinguish healthy and non-healthy eating
   (B) Difficulty withdrawing or eliminating the substance from one's routine
   (C) Continued choice to use the substance despite problems associated with use
   (D) Change in the individuals' tolerance for the substance

26. Spina bifida typically results in which of the following activity limitations?
   (A) Paralysis below the lesion
   (B) Increased likelihood of blood disorders
   (C) Decreased attention span
   (D) Increased motor activity in the lower extremities

27. The *Diagnostic and Statistical Manual of Mental Disorders IV-TR* classifies which type of disorders?
   (A) Mental illness
   (B) Intellectual disability
   (C) Cognitive impairments
   (D) Learning disabilities

28. Clinical supervision is different than managerial supervision in that it
   (A) can only come from CTRSs
   (B) involves mentoring about practice situations and wisdom
   (C) must be sanctioned by NCTRC
   (D) can only occur in clinical facilities

29. According to the Health Protection/Health Promotion model, prescriptive activities help the client
   (A) adjust to multiple medications
   (B) recover from a threat to his/her health
   (C) reintegrate into the community
   (D) alleviate the long-term effects of disability and/or disease

30. In which of the following situations does the individual likely have cataracts?
   (A) The client needs glasses only for near-vision reading.
   (B) The client experiences loss of central vision and has to turn from side to side to see an item directly in front of him.
   (C) The client's vision is blurred and she has trouble seeing things distinctly.
   (D) The client has difficulty seeing at night, often seeing "stars" around bright lights.

31. The *ATRA Standards of Practice* says that quality client assessment is characterized by
   (A) data, action, and response
   (B) leisure interests, health and well-being, and future intentions
   (C) functional abilities that impact leisure involvement
   (D) systematic collection of comprehensive and accurate data to design an individualized treatment plan

32. The most recent and the most preferred national standards for accessibility are contained within the
   (A) Joint Commission's (JCAHO) standards manuals
   (B) *Accessibility Guidelines for America*
   (C) Department of the Interior's park and natural areas guidelines
   (D) Americans with Disabilities Act

33. The CTRS working in a psychiatric facility for adults needs an assessment instrument that has the capability of monitoring clients in the three areas of general performance, individual performance, and group performance. Which of the following published assessment instruments would be MOST suitable?
   (A) Leisure Diagnostic Battery (LDB)
   (B) Comprehensive Evaluation in Recreational Therapy Scale (CERT-Psych)
   (C) Self-Leisure Interest Profile (SLIP)
   (D) Leisure Activities Blank (LAB)

34. Which federal legislation attempts to equalize mental health services with other medical services?
   (A) Mental Health Parity and Addiction Equity Act
   (B) Americans with Disabilities Act
   (C) Equity Healthcare for All Americans Act
   (D) Equal Illness, Equal Healthcare Act

35. After administering the Leisure Diagnostic Battery (LDB), the CTRS scored the client's sub-scales and found that the client had an external locus of control, among other findings. Which of the following client statements would confirm these assessment results?
   (A) "I am a very goal-oriented person."
   (B) "I want you to make that decision for me."
   (C) "I am saving money to go on a vacation next month."
   (D) "I followed up on our conversation and I'm entering that writing contest next week."

36. A clinical CTRS and a community CTRS are conducting a marketing analysis to set-up a joint outpatient TR rehab program. Which statement identifies a factor that would be considered an opportunity to promote this joint venture?
    (A) PT and OT are currently contracting their services in the community
    (B) A private health care company is providing in-home care in the area
    (C) Patient length of stay in inpatient rehabilitation is continuing to decrease
    (D) An ADA survey is presently being conducted in the community

37. When an assessment is norm-referenced, it means that the assessment was/is
    (A) interpreted based on the average scores for that person's peer group
    (B) based on a normal population's average scores
    (C) references using the major texts in the therapeutic recreation literature
    (D) based on scores of normal behavior expected within that developmental life stage

38. A CTRS who works with 3- to 5-year-olds in a preschool program, uses Erikson's Theory of Psychosocial Development to improve the age-appropriateness of his programs. Specifically he teaches the children to
    (A) know when to take action and when to use self-restraint
    (B) play games that require intra-group social interaction skills
    (C) meet their own needs through intrinsically motivated play
    (D) recognize their own strengths and weaknesses

39. Which of the following is a question that addresses content validity?
    (A) How accurately does current content reflect future content?
    (B) How closely related are items on a single assessment?
    (C) How consistent are scores over different parts of the assessment?
    (D) How adequately does the sample of assessment items represent the totality of the content to be measured?

40. A CTRS has been hired as Director of Therapeutic Recreation Services at the local rehabilitation center to start a new program of services and wants to provide the highest quality services available. She reviews which therapeutic recreation standards to assure program compliance?
    (A) *ATRA Standards of Practice*
    (B) Joint Commission (JCAHO) standards
    (C) NCTRC certification standards
    (D) *ATRA Code of Ethics*

41. Which of the following is NOT a benefit of evidence-based practice?
    (A) Helps focus intervention programs on client outcomes
    (B) Improves relative consistency from program to program
    (C) Eliminates need for program evaluation data
    (D) Helps determine content of client assessments

42. The intent of the federal initiative called *Healthy People 2020* is to
    (A) heighten awareness of the overall health of Americans, including those with disabilities
    (B) ensure that Americans understand that eating fast food is the prime predictor of obesity
    (C) monitor the increasing amount of time Americans are spending on exercising
    (D) monitor the effects of low-carbohydrate diets on the obesity of Americans

43. The CTRS had eight four-year-old children who had behavioral problems (like kicking, biting, and spitting on others) compete with each other on two bowling teams. Instead of realizing the children had difficulty interacting in the_____ interaction pattern and having them practice skills at that level, she had them participating in an activity that required a _____ interaction pattern, and thus, the children became aggressive and the activity failed.
    (A) Aggregate, intergroup
    (B) Intraindividual, extraindividual
    (C) Aggregate, interindividual
    (D) Cooperative, competitive

44. Which statement best describes an outcome of completing activity analysis?
    (A) Activities are referenced according to their difficulty
    (B) The amount of time necessary for the client to acquire the skill is determined
    (C) The skills necessary to perform the activity are identified
    (D) The types of adaptations needed by clients are determined

45. In which of the following steps does the CTRS place the client into the most appropriate programs?
    (A) Assessment
    (B) Program planning
    (C) Program implementation
    (D) Program evaluation

46. While teaching adolescents with mild intellectual disability the card game of "Pinochle," the CTRS found that the rules were too complicated for the clients to be successful. The CTRS had inappropriately analyzed and planned the activity in which of the following domains?
    (A) Physical
    (B) Emotional
    (C) Social
    (D) Cognitive

47. All of the following must be protected under the Health Insurance Portability and Accountability Act (HIPAA) 1996 and its updates EXCEPT
    (A) individually identifiable demographic information
    (B) the individual's part, present, or future physical or mental health or condition
    (C) the provision of health care to the individual
    (D) some employment records for some groups of individuals

48. "Frontloading" an activity means that the therapeutic recreation specialist
    (A) plans the activity well in advance of its delivery
    (B) explains the intended outcomes at the beginning of the activity
    (C) places all the materials and props at the front of the room
    (D) uses an icebreaker to facilitate group introductions

49. People who are intrinsically motivated in their leisure tend to
    (A) avoid situations in which they are challenged to demonstrate a certain skill level
    (B) seek challenges equal to their competence
    (C) avoid situations which may result in negative feedback about their performance
    (D) seek situations that are easily accomplished or quickly won

50. During a leisure planning session, a client said, "We used to take lots of vacations as a family, usually for two to three weeks at a time." The CTRS responded, "Tell me more about your vacations." The CTRS was using which of the following communication techniques?
    (A) Probe
    (B) Summarization
    (C) Clarification
    (D) Confrontation

51. The client received burns in a house fire that affected all three layers of skin as well as muscle tissue. She does not feel pain as the nerve fibers and pain receptors have been destroyed. The client's burns are classified as
    (A) intensive
    (B) first-degree
    (C) second-degree
    (D) third-degree

52. Which of the following statements represents the MOST assertive response to the question "Where would you like to eat dinner tonight?"
    (A) "We can go wherever you want"
    (B) "I don't care where we eat, you always choose anyway"
    (C) "I'd like to try that new Italian restaurant by the mall"
    (D) "You should know where I want to eat by now"

53. A CTRS working in a psychiatric facility needs to find information about specific mental illnesses and conditions. Which of the following references would be MOST appropriate?
    (A) *Physicians' Desk Reference*
    (B) *Diagnostic and Statistical Manual-IV-TR*
    (C) *Therapeutic Recreation and the Nature of Disabilities*
    (D) *Comprehensive Accreditation Manual for Behavioral Health Care*

54. The client tends to blame others when something goes wrong and has a difficult time accepting responsibility for her actions. What therapeutic recreation facilitation technique is MOST LIKELY to be helpful for this client?
    (A) Reality therapy
    (B) Anger management
    (C) Resocialization
    (D) Validation therapy

55. A facility that provides comprehensive services for individuals with physical disabilities on an inpatient and outpatient basis is called a
    (A) community mental health center
    (B) physical medicine and rehabilitation center
    (C) sheltered workshop
    (D) homebound program

56. In human anatomy, the scapula performs what function?
    (A) It produces extension and flexion of the upper leg
    (B) It forms the shoulder joint where many bones and muscles originate
    (C) It forms the elbow joint with the humerus proximally
    (D) It serves as the foundation for speech

57. When assessing a child's ability to remain seated during a 30-minute activity, the CTRS would look for which of the following behavioral characteristics?
    (A) Duration of behavior
    (B) Frequency of behavior
    (C) Intensity of behavior
    (D) Rate of the behavior

58. The client, a 10-year-old boy, has been diagnosed with attention-deficit/hyperactivity disorder (ADHD). The CTRS should be aware of which of the following possible effects of ADHD?
    (A) Decreased ability to follow directions
    (B) Blunted feelings
    (C) Above average organizational skills
    (D) Loss of personal sense of identity

59. The Joint Commission (JCAHO) identifies three categories of outcome measures: health status, patient perceptions of care, and client performance outcomes. The CTRS reports on clients' functional improvement, which falls in which of the following outcome categories?
    (A) Health status
    (B) Patient perceptions of care
    (C) Client performance outcomes
    (D) None of the above

60. The symptoms of anorexia nervosa are
    (A) refusal to eat, loss of hair, and frequent vomiting
    (B) binge eating, depression, and weighing constantly
    (C) secretive behavior, hyperactivity, and depression
    (D) growth of fine body hair and loss of 25 percent body weight

61. The MDS 3.0 is an assessment completed for individuals in which type of setting?
    (A) Correctional institutions
    (B) Adult day care centers
    (C) Outpatient rehabilitation programs
    (D) Nursing homes

62. Where is the latissimus dorsi muscle located in the human body?
    (A) leg
    (B) neck
    (C) abdomen
    (D) mid-back

63. Current research has shown that the most common TR services billed for reimbursement include
    (A) client assessment, leisure education, and community re-entry
    (B) client assessment, social skills training, and ADLs
    (C) stress management, group activities, and outpatient services
    (D) values clarification, leisure education, and functional skills training

64. All of the following are considered disadvantages of reviewing medical records instead of interviewing or observing the client EXCEPT
    (A) reducing redundancy for the client
    (B) potential inaccuracy of the data
    (C) limited amount or kinds of data
    (D) reducing personal contact with the client

65. Muscle atrophy is caused by which of the following situations?
(A) Lack of intelligence
(B) Lack of physical activity
(C) Excessive calorie intake compared to energy expenditure
(D) Steroids or human growth hormones

66. After the client assessment has been completed, the next step in the programming process is to
(A) write treatment summaries
(B) analyze activities
(C) identify the problem(s)
(D) develop goals and objectives

67. A client in a substance abuse program, states, "I am looking forward to going home but I worry if I can maintain my sobriety." He is expressing emotions at what level of the Krathwohl's Affective Taxonomy?
(A) Responding
(B) Valuing
(C) Organization
(D) Characterization

68. The purpose of quality improvement activities is to
(A) gather client input into the improvement of programs
(B) increase communication with other members of the treatment team
(C) increase documentation of therapeutic recreation services
(D) improve the effectiveness of client services

69. In which of the four domains does the following statement fall under?
"To increase standing tolerance to 15 minutes"
(A) Cognitive
(B) Affective
(C) Physical
(D) Social

70. Individuals with intellectual disability may have an unrealistic view of "self" for all of the following reasons EXCEPT
(A) lack of exposure to peer groups
(B) parents may be overprotective
(C) difficulty in exploring and testing their own limits
(D) biological changes in the brain

71. A client in a stroke rehabilitation program, states, "I really like to spend time with my family and have two activities planned for this weekend." She is expressing emotions at what level of the Krathwohl's Affective Taxonomy?
(A) Responding
(B) Valuing
(C) Organization
(D) Characterization

72. Spina bifida is a condition in which the spinal column
(A) was injured by traumatic force
(B) is injured posthumously
(C) collapses upon itself
(D) has failed to develop completely

73. Which of the following is NOT a characteristic of "high performance teams" of people working in a health care environment?
(A) Decisions are made by group members
(B) Each person shares in the responsibility for success
(C) Each person works in his or her "work silo"
(D) Responses to requests are timely and efficient

74. Which part of the SOAP progress note is the following statement, "The client lacks adequate knowledge of community resources to be able to function independently."
(A) S – Subjective
(B) O – Objective
(C) A – Assessment
(D) P – Plan

75. Which of the following is an example of "objective" data that may be recorded in a progress note?
(A) The client stated, "I really got a lot out of this program!"
(B) The client's family said that the client was progressing with the outpatient therapy
(C) It appears the client is depressed
(D) The client goes to his room immediately following all sessions

76. According to the Transtheoretical Model, if the client has been walking three miles every other day in order to increase his physical activity levels, he is at what stage of behavior change?
(A) Precontemplation
(B) Contemplation
(C) Preparation
(D) Action

77. Compare the two progress notes written below:
1 Friday, 12/11 - Pt. seemed withdrawn on community outing Friday night

2 Friday, 12/11 - While pt. was attending community outing Friday night, she conversed only once with other pts. for approximately one minute. Pt. remained alone in the corner of the van during transit, and stayed at a separate table during most of the night.

Progress note 2 is the better written than progress note 1 because it
(A) states more consistent information
(B) relies on professional judgments
(C) states behavior rather than conclusions
(D) uses less professional jargon

78. In establishing an environment that embraces multiculturalism, the CTRS would
(A) make sure all ethnic holidays are on the activity calendar
(B) introduce signage that includes both English and Spanish, and possibly French
(C) recognize people's differences while establishing a sense of unity
(D) follow the agency directives with regard to nondiscrimination toward foreigners

79. An insurance carrier's cost control method of paying a prearranged amount for specific service, no matter what the actual cost of those services might be, is called
(A) third-party reimbursement
(B) prospective payment
(C) cost allocation
(D) unit cost

80. The best indication that pain is present is
(A) regression to child-like behaviors
(B) self-report of the client
(C) swelling and redness in the area
(D) a similar occurrence in the past 24 hours

81. The CTRS might use each of the following to assess leisure interests of a client EXCEPT
(A) administering an activity interest inventory to the client
(B) interviewing the client regarding her leisure interests
(C) interviewing the family and/or significant others regarding the client's leisure interests
(D) administering the Functional Independence Measure (FIM)

82. Which of the following is NOT an appropriate question for a cognitive assessment for older adults in long-term care?
(A) What day of the week is it today?
(B) How would you find someone to play cards with while here in the facility?
(C) How often do you talk with family members?
(D) What leisure activities did you like to do before you became a resident here?

83. The CTRS should use which of the following activities to improve the dynamic balance of youth with hearing impairments?
(A) standing on one foot, with arms outstretched
(B) leisure education
(C) running
(D) tumbling

84. What is a primary outcome of completing a task analysis?
(A) Behaviors needed to complete a skill are listed in a teaching sequence
(B) A hierarchy of skills used in an activity are prepared
(C) Each behavioral area exhibited in an activity is compared with one another
(D) The time necessary for intervention is determined

85. While leading a reminiscing group at the long-term care facility, the CTRS was unprepared to console/counsel a patient when he talked about a traumatic and difficult childhood. The CTRS had inappropriately planned and analyzed the activity in which of the following domains?
(A) Physical
(B) Emotional
(C) Social
(D) Cognitive

86. Which of the following documents most directly justify reimbursement for TR services?
(A) Client assessment, treatment protocols, and quality improvement documents
(B) Flow charts and trend analysis
(C) Utilization review documents, treatment protocols, and risk management studies
(D) Policy and procedures manuals

87. The CTRS observes the client's ability to complete a five-minute walking endurance test. What functional behavior is being assessed?
    (A) Cognitive
    (B) Physical
    (C) Social
    (D) Emotional

88. A major advantage to knowing the stages of behavior change in the Transtheoretical Model is that the CTRS can
    (A) provide a variety of leisure resources to the clients
    (B) focus on the concerns at each stage
    (C) motivate clients to learn more leisure activities
    (D) increase attendance at therapeutic recreation programs

89. The first step in a person changing a negative behavior to a positive behavior is
    (A) recognizing the problem behavior
    (B) reappraising the stressors that caused the original incident
    (C) coping with the negative consequences of the original behavior
    (D) believing the negative behavior can be changed

90. The punishment model for corrections may adhere to the following motto
    (A) "An eye for an eye"
    (B) "There is hope for everyone"
    (C) "A stitch in time saves nine"
    (D) "Do unto others as you would have them do unto you"

Practice Test 6

Scoring Sheet

1. Ⓐ Ⓑ Ⓒ Ⓓ   14. Ⓐ Ⓑ Ⓒ Ⓓ   27. Ⓐ Ⓑ Ⓒ Ⓓ   40. Ⓐ Ⓑ Ⓒ Ⓓ

2. Ⓐ Ⓑ Ⓒ Ⓓ   15. Ⓐ Ⓑ Ⓒ Ⓓ   28. Ⓐ Ⓑ Ⓒ Ⓓ   41. Ⓐ Ⓑ Ⓒ Ⓓ

3. Ⓐ Ⓑ Ⓒ Ⓓ   16. Ⓐ Ⓑ Ⓒ Ⓓ   29. Ⓐ Ⓑ Ⓒ Ⓓ   42. Ⓐ Ⓑ Ⓒ Ⓓ

4. Ⓐ Ⓑ Ⓒ Ⓓ   17. Ⓐ Ⓑ Ⓒ Ⓓ   30. Ⓐ Ⓑ Ⓒ Ⓓ   43. Ⓐ Ⓑ Ⓒ Ⓓ

5. Ⓐ Ⓑ Ⓒ Ⓓ   18. Ⓐ Ⓑ Ⓒ Ⓓ   31. Ⓐ Ⓑ Ⓒ Ⓓ   44. Ⓐ Ⓑ Ⓒ Ⓓ

6. Ⓐ Ⓑ Ⓒ Ⓓ   19. Ⓐ Ⓑ Ⓒ Ⓓ   32. Ⓐ Ⓑ Ⓒ Ⓓ   45. Ⓐ Ⓑ Ⓒ Ⓓ

7. Ⓐ Ⓑ Ⓒ Ⓓ   20. Ⓐ Ⓑ Ⓒ Ⓓ   33. Ⓐ Ⓑ Ⓒ Ⓓ   46. Ⓐ Ⓑ Ⓒ Ⓓ

8. Ⓐ Ⓑ Ⓒ Ⓓ   21. Ⓐ Ⓑ Ⓒ Ⓓ   34. Ⓐ Ⓑ Ⓒ Ⓓ   47. Ⓐ Ⓑ Ⓒ Ⓓ

9. Ⓐ Ⓑ Ⓒ Ⓓ   22. Ⓐ Ⓑ Ⓒ Ⓓ   35. Ⓐ Ⓑ Ⓒ Ⓓ   48. Ⓐ Ⓑ Ⓒ Ⓓ

10. Ⓐ Ⓑ Ⓒ Ⓓ   23. Ⓐ Ⓑ Ⓒ Ⓓ   36. Ⓐ Ⓑ Ⓒ Ⓓ   49. Ⓐ Ⓑ Ⓒ Ⓓ

11. Ⓐ Ⓑ Ⓒ Ⓓ   24. Ⓐ Ⓑ Ⓒ Ⓓ   37. Ⓐ Ⓑ Ⓒ Ⓓ   50. Ⓐ Ⓑ Ⓒ Ⓓ

12. Ⓐ Ⓑ Ⓒ Ⓓ   25. Ⓐ Ⓑ Ⓒ Ⓓ   38. Ⓐ Ⓑ Ⓒ Ⓓ   51. Ⓐ Ⓑ Ⓒ Ⓓ

13. Ⓐ Ⓑ Ⓒ Ⓓ   26. Ⓐ Ⓑ Ⓒ Ⓓ   39. Ⓐ Ⓑ Ⓒ Ⓓ   52. Ⓐ Ⓑ Ⓒ Ⓓ

53. Ⓐ Ⓑ Ⓒ Ⓓ   66. Ⓐ Ⓑ Ⓒ Ⓓ   79. Ⓐ Ⓑ Ⓒ Ⓓ

54. Ⓐ Ⓑ Ⓒ Ⓓ   67. Ⓐ Ⓑ Ⓒ Ⓓ   80. Ⓐ Ⓑ Ⓒ Ⓓ

55. Ⓐ Ⓑ Ⓒ Ⓓ   68. Ⓐ Ⓑ Ⓒ Ⓓ   81. Ⓐ Ⓑ Ⓒ Ⓓ

56. Ⓐ Ⓑ Ⓒ Ⓓ   69. Ⓐ Ⓑ Ⓒ Ⓓ   82. Ⓐ Ⓑ Ⓒ Ⓓ

57. Ⓐ Ⓑ Ⓒ Ⓓ   70. Ⓐ Ⓑ Ⓒ Ⓓ   83. Ⓐ Ⓑ Ⓒ Ⓓ

58. Ⓐ Ⓑ Ⓒ Ⓓ   71. Ⓐ Ⓑ Ⓒ Ⓓ   84. Ⓐ Ⓑ Ⓒ Ⓓ

59. Ⓐ Ⓑ Ⓒ Ⓓ   72. Ⓐ Ⓑ Ⓒ Ⓓ   85. Ⓐ Ⓑ Ⓒ Ⓓ

60. Ⓐ Ⓑ Ⓒ Ⓓ   73. Ⓐ Ⓑ Ⓒ Ⓓ   86. Ⓐ Ⓑ Ⓒ Ⓓ

61. Ⓐ Ⓑ Ⓒ Ⓓ   74. Ⓐ Ⓑ Ⓒ Ⓓ   87. Ⓐ Ⓑ Ⓒ Ⓓ

62. Ⓐ Ⓑ Ⓒ Ⓓ   75. Ⓐ Ⓑ Ⓒ Ⓓ   88. Ⓐ Ⓑ Ⓒ Ⓓ

63. Ⓐ Ⓑ Ⓒ Ⓓ   76. Ⓐ Ⓑ Ⓒ Ⓓ   89. Ⓐ Ⓑ Ⓒ Ⓓ

64. Ⓐ Ⓑ Ⓒ Ⓓ   77. Ⓐ Ⓑ Ⓒ Ⓓ   90. Ⓐ Ⓑ Ⓒ Ⓓ

65. Ⓐ Ⓑ Ⓒ Ⓓ   78. Ⓐ Ⓑ Ⓒ Ⓓ

Practice Test 6

Scoring Key

Foundational Knowledge

2. C	18. B	34. A	51. D	65. B	80. B
4. B	25. A	38. A	53. B	70. D	83. D
7. B	27. A	42. A	56. B	72. D	88. B
12. B	30. C	47. D	60. D	76. D	89. A
16. A	32. D	49. B	62. D	78. C	90. A

Practice of TR/RT

1. A	19. B	33. B	46. D	61. D	75. D
3. D	21. A	35. B	48. B	64. A	77. C
6. B	22. C	37. A	50. A	66. C	81. D
8. D	24. A	39. D	52. C	67. D	82. C
10. D	26. A	41. C	54. A	69. C	84. A
14. C	29. B	43. A	57. A	71. B	85. B
17. D	31. D	44. C	58. A	74. C	87. B

Organization of TR/RT

9. D	13. B	23. B	55. B	68. D	79. B
11. D	20. B	45. A	63. A	73. C	86. A

Advancement of the Profession

5. A	15. D	28. B	36. C	40. A	59. C

PRACTICE TEST 6

Record Your Scores Here

Foundational Knowledge	_____ / 30 =	_____ %
Practice of TR/RT	_____ / 42 =	_____ %
Organization of TR/RT	_____ / 12 =	_____ %
Advancement of the Profession	_____ / 6 =	_____ %

Total Score = _____ /90

Total Percent = _____ %

TEST SUMMARIES

WARM-UP ITEMS

Foundational Knowledge _____ / 43 = _____ %
Practice of TR/RT _____ / 73 = _____ %
Organization of TR/RT _____ / 31 = _____ %
Advancement of the Profession _____ / 13 = _____ %

Total Score = _____ /160
Total Percent = _____ %

PRACTICE TEST 1

Foundational Knowledge _____ / 30 = _____ %
Practice of TR/RT _____ / 42 = _____ %
Organization of TR/RT _____ / 12 = _____ %
Advancement of the Profession _____ / 6 = _____ %

Total Score = _____ /90
Total Percent = _____ %

PRACTICE TEST 2

Foundational Knowledge _____ / 30 = _____ %
Practice of TR/RT _____ / 42 = _____ %
Organization of TR/RT _____ / 12 = _____ %
Advancement of the Profession _____ / 6 = _____ %

Total Score = _____ /90
Total Percent = _____ %

PRACTICE TEST 3

Foundational Knowledge _____ / 30 = _____ %
Practice of TR/RT _____ / 42 = _____ %
Organization of TR/RT _____ / 12 = _____ %
Advancement of the Profession _____ / 6 = _____ %

Total Score = _____ /90
Total Percent = _____ %

PRACTICE TEST 4

Foundational Knowledge _____ / 30 = _____ %
Practice of TR/RT _____ / 42 = _____ %
Organization of TR/RT _____ / 12 = _____ %
Advancement of the Profession _____ / 6 = _____ %

Total Score = _____ /90
Total Percent = _____ %

ce

PRACTICE TEST 5

Foundational Knowledge _____/ 30 = _____ %
Practice of TR/RT _____/ 42 = _____ %
Organization of TR/RT _____/ 12 = _____ %
Advancement of the Profession _____/ 6 = _____ %

Total Score = _____ /90
Total Percent = _____ %

PRACTICE TEST 6

Foundational Knowledge _____/ 30 = _____ %
Practice of TR/RT _____/ 42 = _____ %
Organization of TR/RT _____/ 12 = _____ %
Advancement of the Profession _____/ 6 = _____ %

Total Score = _____ /90
Total Percent = _____ %

AREAS OF STRENGTH:

_____
_____
_____
_____
_____
_____
_____
_____

AREAS FOR FURTHER STUDY:

_____
_____
_____
_____
_____
_____
_____
_____